Type 2 Diabetes Cookbook
Beginner's Quick & Easy Recipes for Delicious Diabetes Diets

300 Healthy

<u>Breakfasts</u>

for

Diabetic Wellness in 30 Minutes or Less

By

Lily Anders

Copyright Page

Ace East Publishing LLC
1401 21st Street
Suite R
Sacramento, CA 95811

ISBN: **978-1-963939-86-6**

Second Edition

ACE EAST PUBLISHING

Disclaimer Page

This cookbook is crafted to offer insightful information and recipes for those interested in managing Type 2 Diabetes through dietary choices. It is important to recognize that the authors and the publisher are not healthcare professionals. The suggestions and recipes contained within this book are not meant to replace professional medical advice, diagnoses, or treatments. Should you have any healthcare-related questions or concerns, particularly relating to Type 2 Diabetes management, we strongly advise consulting with your doctor or a qualified healthcare provider.

The culinary experiences and recommendations shared in this book stem from extensive research and the personal journey of exploring dietary approaches to Type 2 Diabetes management. These narratives and suggestions are intended for educational and motivational purposes only, aiming to enhance understanding and inspire positive lifestyle changes, not to serve as direct medical or nutritional prescriptions.

The author(s) and publisher expressly disclaim any liability for any adverse effects arising directly or indirectly from the use and application of the information contained in this cookbook. Moreover, given the specificity and medical relevance of the content, certain topics and dietary advice may not be suitable for all readers. It is advisable for caregivers and adults to review the content before sharing it with minors or individuals with particular sensitivities or health concerns.

In cases of medical emergencies or for immediate assistance with health issues, please reach out to a trusted healthcare professional or dial the emergency services number available in your locality.

The Entire Type 2 Diabetes Cookbook Series

Dive into a culinary revolution with the ***"Type 2 Diabetes Cookbook Series: Beginner's Quick & Easy Recipes for Delicious Diabetes Diets – 300 Health-Boosting Savory Meals for Diabetic Wellness in 30 Minutes or Less."***

Spread across six essential volumes – Breakfast, Lunch, Dinner, Desserts, Snacks, and Sauces, Dips, & Dressings – this series is your passport to a world where managing Type 2 Diabetes meets delicious innovation.

Each book is a treasure trove of hundreds of recipes, marrying the precision of nutritional science with the flair of culinary art. Designed for those on a diabetic diet, these recipes promise to transform your meals from bland to blissful without sacrificing flavor or health. Every dish, from energizing breakfasts to indulgent desserts, comes alive through vivid, full-color photographs, accompanied by foolproof instructions, cooking times, detailed ingredient lists, serving suggestions, and handy conversion charts.

But the journey doesn't end with tantalizing meals. These cookbooks are gateways to mastering diabetes management, offering insights into blood sugar balance, insulin functionality, and the art of carb counting. They stand as pillars of empowerment and knowledge, guiding you through the culinary and health aspects of diabetes with ease and enjoyment.

Embrace these cookbooks as more than mere collections of recipes; see them as companions in your journey toward diabetic wellness, bringing confidence, pleasure, and a burst of flavors into your daily life. Step into a world where managing diabetes is synonymous with culinary discovery and dietary joy. Welcome to your new kitchen adventure!

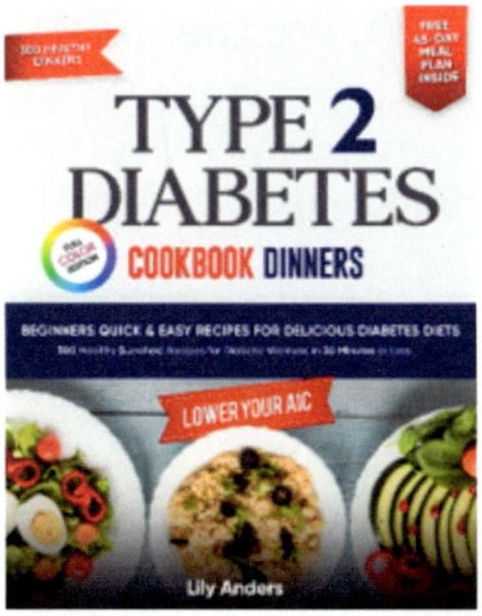
FREE 45-DAY MEAL PLAN INSIDE
TYPE 2
DIABETES
COOKBOOK DINNERS
BEGINNERS QUICK & EASY RECIPES FOR DELICIOUS DIABETES DIETS
LOWER YOUR A1C
Lily Anders

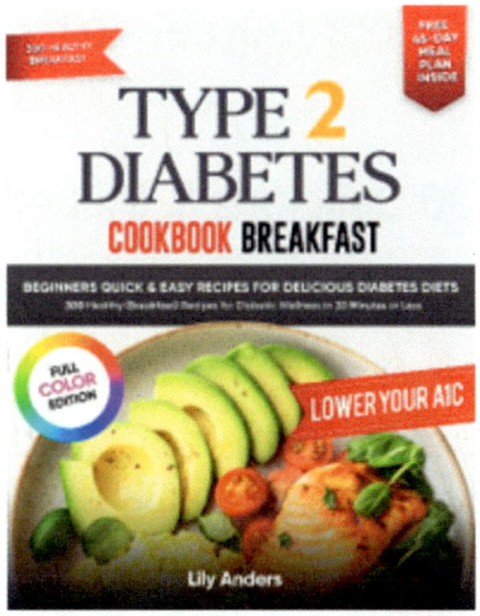
FREE 45-DAY MEAL PLAN INSIDE
TYPE 2
DIABETES
COOKBOOK BREAKFAST
BEGINNERS QUICK & EASY RECIPES FOR DELICIOUS DIABETES DIETS
FULL COLOR EDITION
LOWER YOUR A1C
Lily Anders

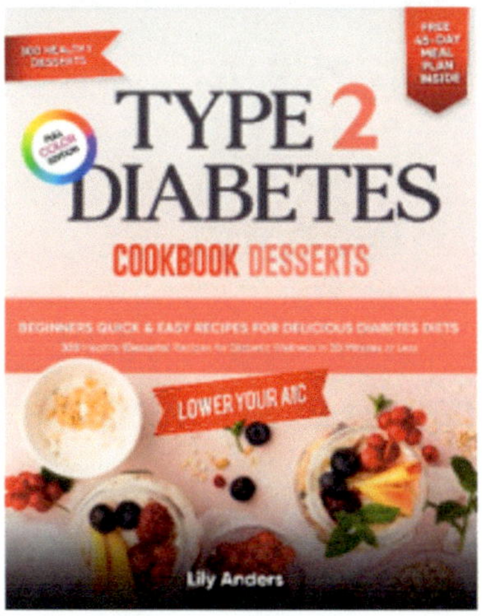
FREE 45-DAY MEAL PLAN INSIDE
TYPE 2
DIABETES
COOKBOOK DESSERTS
BEGINNERS QUICK & EASY RECIPES FOR DELICIOUS DIABETES DIETS
LOWER YOUR A1C
Lily Anders

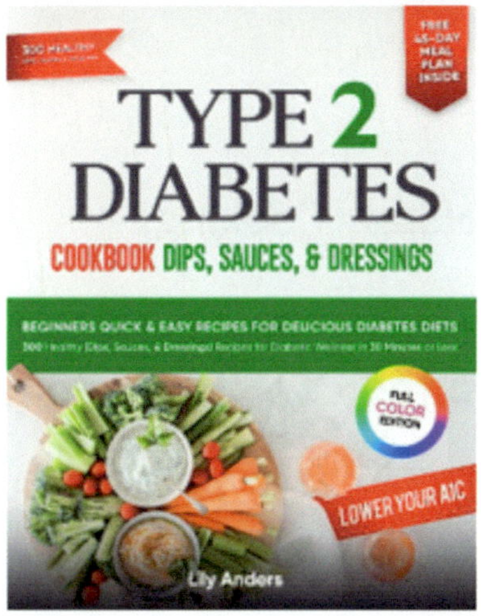
FREE 45-DAY MEAL PLAN INSIDE
TYPE 2
DIABETES
COOKBOOK DIPS, SAUCES, & DRESSINGS
BEGINNERS QUICK & EASY RECIPES FOR DELICIOUS DIABETES DIETS
FULL COLOR EDITION
LOWER YOUR A1C
Lily Anders

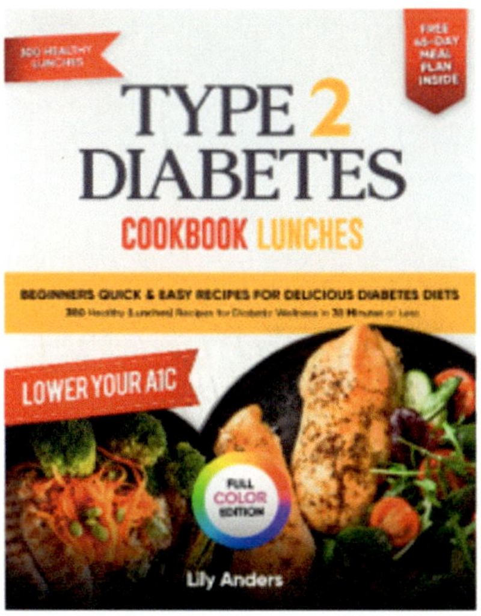
FREE 45-DAY MEAL PLAN INSIDE
TYPE 2
DIABETES
COOKBOOK LUNCHES
BEGINNERS QUICK & EASY RECIPES FOR DELICIOUS DIABETES DIETS
LOWER YOUR A1C
FULL COLOR EDITION
Lily Anders

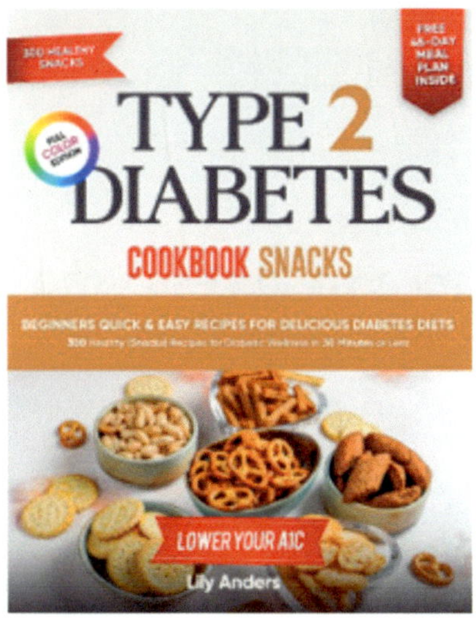
FREE 45-DAY MEAL PLAN INSIDE
TYPE 2
DIABETES
COOKBOOK SNACKS
BEGINNERS QUICK & EASY RECIPES FOR DELICIOUS DIABETES DIETS
LOWER YOUR A1C
Lily Anders

Here's My Promise to You!

To jumpstart your journey toward healthier eating, here are the remaining

Listing of 200 Delicious & Diabetes-Friendly Breakfast Recipes!

That's right—you now have access to a treasure trove of 200 additional diabetic recipes designed to help you enjoy flavorful, balanced meals while managing your blood sugar with confidence. These Breakfast recipes will inspire you to create satisfying, nutritious meals with ease.

☞ CLICK THE LINK OR SCAN THE QR CODE TO DOWNLOAD YOUR FREE RECIPE COLLECTION!

Enjoy, and Happy Cooking!

The journey to better health starts with the right food choices, and this cookbook and it is here to support you every step of the way.

Thank you for trusting this guide, and here's to a flavorful, balanced, and empowered approach to managing Type 2 Diabetes!

You've got this! ☐☐✨

<<Click here to access your 45-day meal plan>>
https://acrobat.adobe.com/id/urn:aaid:sc:VA6C2:448a7fa7-ffcd-4919-9d29-1c8e6bee62e9

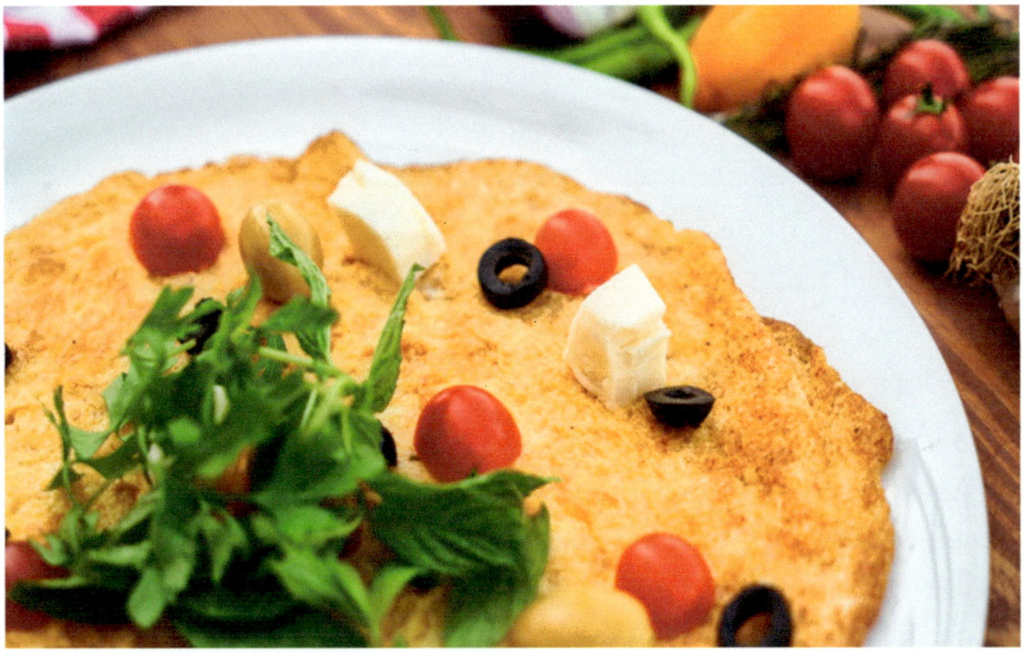

1. Vegetable Omelet

Prep.Time: 5 min	Cook Time: 5-7 min	Serving: 1	Beverage pairing: Green Tea

Ingredients:

- 2 large eggs
- 1/4 cup diced bell peppers (any color)
- 1/4 cup diced onions
- 1/4 cup diced tomatoes
- 1/4 cup chopped spinach
- 1/4 teaspoon black pepper
- 1/4 teaspoon salt (optional)
- 1 teaspoon olive oil

Preparation:

- In a mixing bowl, beat the eggs until well mixed.
- Add diced bell peppers, onions, tomatoes, chopped spinach, black pepper, and salt (if using) to the eggs. Mix well.
- Heat olive oil in a non-stick skillet over medium heat.
- Pour the egg mixture into the skillet and spread it evenly.
- Cook for 2-3 minutes until the edges start to set.
- Carefully flip the omelette and cook for another 2-3 minutes until cooked through.
- Slide the omelette onto a plate and fold it in half.

Nutrient Facts (per serving):

- Calories: 180
- Carbohydrates: 6g
- Fat: 12g
- Protein: 12g

Table of Contents

Copyright Page....2

Disclaimer Page....3

The Entire Type 2 Diabetes Cookbook Series....4

Here's My Promise to You!....6

INTRODUCTION....13

Starting the Day Right with Type 2 Diabetes....13

Chapter 1....15

Understanding Type 2 Diabetes: A Breakfast Perspective....15

Why Mornings Matter More Than You Think....15

Type 2 Diabetes Is Not the Same for Everyone....15

The Role of Breakfast in Long-Term Consistency....16

Chapter 2....17

Blood Sugar and the Morning Window....17

The Morning Blood Sugar Response....17

Creating Stability Instead of Spikes....17

The Cost of Skipping Breakfast....17

Working With Your Body's Natural Rhythm....18

Chapter 3....19

Carbohydrates at Breakfast Without Fear....19

Why Carbohydrates Matter in the Morning....19

Quality Over Elimination....19

Portion Awareness Without Obsession....20

Pairing for Balance....20

Building Confidence Through Experience....20

Chapter 4....22

Smart Breakfast Shopping....22

Navigating the Breakfast Aisles with Confidence....22

Choosing Carbohydrates Wisely....22

Protein and Healthy Fat Essentials....22

Planning for Convenience....23

Making Breakfast Shopping Sustainable 23
Chapter 5 24
Pantry and Prep for Easy Mornings 24
Stocking a Breakfast-Friendly Pantry 24
Refrigerated Essentials for Balanced Breakfasts 24
Simple Prep Strategies That Save Time 24
Reducing Decision Fatigue 25
Creating a Supportive Morning Environment 25
Chapter 6 26
Portion Awareness at Breakfast 26
Why Portions Matter in the Morning 26
Understanding Breakfast Portions Without Measuring Everything 26
Common Breakfast Portion Pitfalls 26
Finding What Works for You 27
Building Confidence Through Routine 27
Bringing It All Together 28
Let these recipes support your mornings, nourish your body, and remind you that managing Type 2 Diabetes can be both practical and satisfying. 28
1. Vegetable Omelet 29
2. Greek Yogurt Berry Bowl 30
3. Quinoa Breakfast Porridge 31
4. Whole Grain Pancakes with Berries 32
5.Avocado and Poached Egg Toast 33
6. Cottage Cheese Parfait 34
7.Sweet Potato and Turkey Hash 35
8.Chia Seed Pudding 36
9. Spinach and Feta Breakfast Wrap 37
10. Almond Butter Banana Smoothie 38
11. Egg Muffins with Veggies 39
12. Cauliflower and Cheese Breakfast Casserole 40
13. Blueberry Almond Overnight Oats 41
14. Turkey Sausage and Veggie Skillet 42

15. Mango Coconut Chia Pudding 43
16. Peanut Butter Banana Sandwich 44
17. Zucchini and Tomato Frittata 45
18. Ricotta and Berry Stuffed French Toast 46
19. Quiche with Spinach and Mushrooms 47
20. Cherry Almond Breakfast Bowl 48
21. Smoked Salmon and Cream Cheese Bagel 49
22. Apple Cinnamon Quinoa Bowl 50
23. Scrambled Tofu with Tomatoes and Spinach 51
24. Kiwi and Kale Smoothie 52
25. Caprese Avocado Toast 53
26. Breakfast Burrito with Black Beans and Salsa 54
27. Pomegranate and Pistachio Yogurt Parfait 55
28. Oat Bran and Berry Muffins 56
29. Chicken Apple Sausage Breakfast Skillet 57
30. Pear and Walnut Overnight Oats 58
31. Mediterranean Egg White Wrap 59
32. Raspberry Almond Chia Smoothie 60
33. Turkey Bacon and Egg Muffin 61
34. Cinnamon Raisin French Toast 62
35. Veggie-loaded Breakfast Quesadilla 63
36. Banana Nut Quinoa Muffins 64
37. Green Tea Matcha Smoothie 65
38. Spinach and Mushroom Breakfast Burrito 66
39. Coconut Almond Granola with Yogurt 67
40. Orange Cranberry Overnight Oats 68
41. Broccoli and Cheddar Egg Cups 69
42. Chocolate Protein Pancakes 70
43. Mixed Berry Quinoa Parfait 71
44. Mexican Shakshuka 72
45. Apple Pecan Breakfast Couscous 73
46. Avocado and Black Bean Breakfast Bowl 74

47. Vanilla Almond Chia Pudding....75
48. Almond Joy Smoothie Bowl....76
49. Turkey Sausage Breakfast Casserole....77
50. Peach Cobbler Overnight Oats....78
51. Blueberry Lemon Ricotta Pancakes....82
52. Veggie and Feta Breakfast Wrap....83
53. Tomato Basil Quiche....84
54. Mango Pineapple Smoothie....85
55. Caramelized Onion and Mushroom Omelette....86
56. Cranberry Orange Scones....87
57. Southwest Tofu Scramble....88
58. Raspberry Coconut Chia Pudding....89
59. Turkey and Veggie Breakfast Burrito....90
60. Greek Yogurt and Berry Smoothie....91
61. Almond Flour Banana Bread....92
62. Spinach and Tomato Breakfast Pizza....93
63. Hazelnut Mocha Protein Smoothie....94
64. Quinoa and Kale Breakfast Bowl....95
65. Blackberry Walnut Overnight Oats....96
66. Asparagus and Goat Cheese Frittata....97
67. Pumpkin Spice Chia Seed Pudding....98
68. Banana Walnut Breakfast Cookies....99
69. Mediterranean Breakfast Panini....100
70. Strawberry Cheesecake Parfait....101
71. Sweet Potato and Kale Breakfast Skillet....102
72. Chocolate Peanut Butter Protein Pancakes....103
73. Egg and Spinach Breakfast Sandwich....104
74. Cinnamon Apple Quinoa Bowl....105
75. Southwest Breakfast Casserole....106
76. Blueberry Almond Butter Smoothie....107
77. Tomato Basil Avocado Toast....108
78. Pineapple Coconut Chia Pudding....109

79. Turkey Sausage and Sweet Potato Hash....110
80. Raspberry Chocolate Chip Muffins....111
81. Veggie and Hummus Breakfast Wrap....112
82. Vanilla Fig Protein Smoothie....113
83. Apple Cider Quinoa Porridge....114
84. Caprese Egg Cups....115
85. Pecan Pie Overnight Oats....116
86. Breakfast Stuffed Bell Peppers....117
87. Mango Basil Yogurt Parfait....118
88. Lemon Poppy Seed Pancakes....119
89. Greek Omelette with Olives and Feta....120
90. Blueberry Banana Breakfast Burrito....121
91. Coconut Mango Smoothie Bowl....122
92. Pumpkin Walnut Breakfast Quinoa....123
93. Spinach and Artichoke Quiche....124
94. Almond Joy Chia Pudding....125
95. Turkey and Cranberry Breakfast Sandwich....126
96. Chocolate Raspberry Protein Pancakes....127
97. Avocado and Cherry Tomato Bagel....128
98. Peach Almond Breakfast Couscous....129
99. Broccoli and Cheddar Breakfast Muffins....130
100. Kiwi Lime Overnight Oats....131

INTRODUCTION

Being diagnosed with Type 2 Diabetes often changes the way you look at food, but nowhere is that shift felt more strongly than at breakfast.

For many people, mornings suddenly become uncertain. Foods that once felt routine, toast, cereal, and fruit, now raise questions. You may find yourself standing in the kitchen, wondering what is "safe," what is "off-limits," and whether skipping breakfast might be easier than risking a mistake. What was once a simple start to the day can feel confusing, restrictive, and stressful.

This book was written for that moment.

The Type 2 Diabetes Cookbook: Breakfast is designed to remove uncertainty from your mornings and replace it with clarity, confidence, and practical solutions. Rather than relying on extreme dietary rules or complicated nutritional theories, this book focuses on real breakfasts made for real people, meals you can prepare quickly, enjoy fully, and trust to support your diabetic wellness.

Starting the Day Right with Type 2 Diabetes

Breakfast plays a unique role in managing Type 2 Diabetes. After an overnight fast, your body is particularly sensitive to the foods you eat. The choices you make in the morning can influence your blood sugar stability, energy levels, and appetite for the rest of the day. A balanced breakfast can help establish steady momentum, while an imbalanced one may lead to spikes, crashes, and increased cravings later on.

The good news is that a diabetes-friendly breakfast does not have to be boring, time-consuming, or restrictive.

Inside this book, you will find **300 carefully crafted breakfast recipes**, all designed to be prepared in **30 minutes or less**. These recipes emphasize balance, pairing carbohydrates with protein, fiber, and healthy fats to support steady blood sugar levels without sacrificing flavor or satisfaction. From warm breakfasts to grab-and-go options, each recipe is designed for busy mornings and long-term consistency.

This cookbook is not about perfection. It is about progress, practicality, and peace of mind.

You will not be asked to eliminate entire food groups or follow rigid rules. Instead, you will learn how to make thoughtful breakfast choices that work within your lifestyle. Whether you are newly diagnosed or have been managing Type 2 Diabetes for years, this book offers structure without pressure and guidance without judgment.

To help you get the most out of this cookbook, a **free 45-day breakfast meal plan** is included. This plan is optional but designed to reduce decision fatigue, making it easier to stay consistent and build confidence in your choices.

Most importantly, this book is meant to reassure you that managing Type 2 Diabetes does not mean giving up enjoyment or starting each day with anxiety. Breakfast can once again become a nourishing, satisfying, and supportive part of your routine.

You do not have to fear the morning.
You do not have to guess.
And you do not have to navigate this alone.

Welcome to a healthier, more confident start to your day.

Chapter 1

Understanding Type 2 Diabetes: A Breakfast Perspective

Type 2 Diabetes is often described in medical terms, such as blood glucose levels, insulin resistance, and metabolic function. While these concepts are important, understanding Type 2 Diabetes does not require a medical background. What matters most is knowing how your body responds to food, especially at the start of the day.

At its core, Type 2 Diabetes occurs when the body has difficulty using insulin effectively. Insulin is a hormone that helps move glucose, or sugar, from the bloodstream into the cells where it can be used for energy. When insulin does not work as efficiently as it should, glucose remains in the bloodstream longer than intended, causing blood sugar levels to rise.

For many individuals, this process develops gradually. The body may still produce insulin, but the cells become less responsive to it, a condition known as insulin resistance. Over time, this makes blood sugar management more challenging, particularly when meals are unbalanced or poorly timed.

Why Mornings Matter More Than You Think

After an overnight fast, your body enters the day in a unique metabolic state. Blood sugar levels are typically lower, but the body is also more sensitive to the foods you consume. This means that breakfast choices can have a stronger impact than meals eaten later in the day.

A breakfast that is high in refined carbohydrates and low in protein or fiber may cause blood sugar levels to rise quickly, followed by an energy crash. This pattern often leads to increased hunger, cravings, and overeating later in the day. For individuals managing Type 2 Diabetes, these fluctuations can make blood sugar control feel unpredictable and frustrating.

On the other hand, a well-balanced breakfast helps establish stability. When carbohydrates are paired with protein, fiber, and healthy fats, glucose is absorbed more slowly. This steady release of energy supports better blood sugar balance, improved focus, and sustained fullness throughout the morning.

Type 2 Diabetes Is Not the Same for Everyone

It is important to recognize that Type 2 Diabetes does not affect everyone in the same way. Factors such as genetics, lifestyle, activity level, stress, and sleep all influence how the body processes food. What works well for one person may need a slight adjustment for another.

This is why rigid, one-size-fits-all breakfast rules often fail.

Rather than prescribing strict limitations, this book focuses on patterns that consistently support diabetic wellness. These patterns emphasize balance, portion awareness, and food quality, principles that can be adapted to individual preferences and routines.

The Role of Breakfast in Long-Term Consistency

Managing Type 2 Diabetes is not about isolated meals; it is about building habits that are sustainable over time. Breakfast plays a foundational role in that process because it sets the tone for the rest of the day.

When breakfast feels manageable and enjoyable, it becomes easier to maintain consistency. Consistent mornings lead to fewer mid-morning crashes, better meal choices later in the day, and reduced decision fatigue. Over time, this consistency supports healthier blood sugar patterns and a more positive relationship with food.

This book does not promise instant results or perfect control. Instead, it provides a practical framework for starting each day with intention and confidence. By understanding how Type 2 Diabetes interacts with morning nutrition, you gain the ability to make informed choices without fear or confusion.

In the next chapter, we will explore how blood sugar behaves specifically in the morning hours and why certain breakfast combinations work better than others.

Chapter 2

Blood Sugar and the Morning Window

The hours immediately after waking represent a unique period for blood sugar management. What you eat in the morning does more than satisfy hunger. It influences how your body responds to food, energy demands, and insulin throughout the day.

After several hours without food, the body is in a fasted state. During this time, the liver releases stored glucose to maintain normal blood sugar levels. When breakfast is introduced, the body must quickly adjust to the new energy input. For individuals managing Type 2 Diabetes, this transition is especially important.

The Morning Blood Sugar Response

In the morning, insulin sensitivity can vary. Some people experience heightened sensitivity, while others notice a stronger blood sugar response to carbohydrates. This variability is one reason breakfast often feels unpredictable.

A breakfast that contains mostly refined carbohydrates, such as sugary cereals or white bread, may cause blood sugar levels to rise rapidly. Without adequate protein, fiber, or fat to slow digestion, glucose enters the bloodstream quickly. This can result in a sharp spike, followed by a sudden drop, leaving you feeling tired, hungry, or unfocused.

These swings are not a sign of failure. They are a signal that the body needs better balance.

Creating Stability Instead of Spikes

A balanced breakfast helps smooth the transition from fasting to fueling. When carbohydrates are paired with protein and fiber, digestion slows, and glucose is released more gradually. This steadier rise in blood sugar supports consistent energy and reduces the likelihood of mid-morning crashes.

For example, pairing whole grains with eggs, yogurt, or nuts helps create a more stable response than carbohydrates alone. Adding fiber-rich fruits or vegetables further supports blood sugar control without eliminating carbohydrates altogether.

The goal is not to remove carbohydrates from breakfast. The goal is to choose combinations that work with your body rather than against it.

The Cost of Skipping Breakfast

Many people managing Type 2 Diabetes choose to skip breakfast out of fear or uncertainty. While this may seem like a safe option, it can create unintended challenges.

Skipping breakfast often leads to increased hunger later in the day, making portion control more difficult at lunch or dinner. It may also contribute to blood sugar fluctuations as the body compensates for prolonged fasting. Over time, this pattern can increase stress around food choices and disrupt consistency.

Eating a balanced breakfast, even a simple one, provides structure and predictability. This structure makes it easier to maintain healthy patterns throughout the day.

Working With Your Body's Natural Rhythm

Your body follows daily rhythms that influence digestion, hormone release, and energy use. Morning meals play a key role in signaling that the day has begun and that fuel is available.

When breakfast is consistent and balanced, the body responds with improved regulation. Energy levels feel steadier, focus improves, and cravings are often reduced. These effects support better decision-making later in the day, reinforcing a positive cycle.

This book emphasizes breakfasts that respect this rhythm. Meals are designed to be satisfying without being heavy and nourishing without being complicated.

In the next chapter, we will focus specifically on carbohydrates at breakfast, how to approach them without fear, and how portion awareness can make a meaningful difference.

Chapter 3

Carbohydrates at Breakfast Without Fear

For many people managing Type 2 Diabetes, carbohydrates become the most confusing part of breakfast. Messages from diet trends, online forums, and well-meaning advice often suggest that carbohydrates should be avoided entirely. As a result, fear replaces understanding, and breakfast becomes restrictive rather than supportive.

The truth is simpler and far more encouraging.

Carbohydrates are not the enemy. The challenge lies in how they are chosen, portioned, and paired.

Why Carbohydrates Matter in the Morning

Carbohydrates are a primary source of energy for the body and brain. In the morning, when the body is transitioning out of a fasted state, carbohydrates can play a useful role in restoring energy and focus.

Problems arise when carbohydrates are consumed alone or in excess. Refined carbohydrates, such as white bread or sugary cereals, are digested quickly and can cause blood sugar levels to rise rapidly. Without protein, fiber, or fat to slow this process, the result is often a spike followed by a crash.

Balanced carbohydrates, on the other hand, provide steady fuel. When paired properly, they support both blood sugar stability and satisfaction.

Quality Over Elimination

Eliminating carbohydrates entirely is neither necessary nor sustainable for most people. Instead, focusing on carbohydrate quality makes a meaningful difference.

Whole grains, fruits, and vegetables contain fiber, which slows digestion and helps regulate blood sugar. These carbohydrates behave differently in the body than highly processed foods. Choosing whole, minimally processed options allows carbohydrates to remain part of a diabetes-friendly breakfast.

For example, whole oats paired with protein-rich yogurt create a very different blood sugar response than sweetened instant oatmeal eaten alone. The combination matters as much as the ingredient itself.

Portion Awareness Without Obsession

Portion size plays a significant role in how carbohydrates affect blood sugar. Even high-quality carbohydrates can create challenges when portions are too large.

This does not require strict counting or constant measurement. Instead, it involves awareness. Understanding what a reasonable portion looks like helps maintain balance without creating stress.

Breakfast portions should feel satisfying, not excessive. When meals are balanced, smaller portions often feel more filling because digestion slows and energy lasts longer.

Pairing for Balance

One of the most effective ways to manage carbohydrates at breakfast is through thoughtful pairing.

Protein helps slow digestion and promotes fullness. Healthy fats add satisfaction and help stabilize energy levels. Fiber further reduces the speed at which glucose enters the bloodstream.

When carbohydrates are paired with one or more of these elements, the overall blood sugar response becomes gentler and more predictable.

A slice of whole-grain toast paired with eggs and avocado, for example, supports blood sugar balance more effectively than toast alone. A smoothie that includes protein and fiber behaves differently from one made only with fruit.

These combinations allow carbohydrates to work in harmony with the body.

Building Confidence Through Experience

Fear often comes from uncertainty. As you begin to observe how your body responds to different breakfast combinations, confidence grows.

This book encourages experimentation within a structured framework. Recipes are designed to demonstrate balance in action, helping you see that carbohydrates can be included without negative outcomes.

Over time, patterns become clearer. Certain combinations will work especially well for you, while others may need adjustment. This is a normal part of learning to manage Type 2 Diabetes in a way that fits your life.

In the next chapter, we will shift focus to practical preparation, including how to shop for breakfast ingredients and set up your kitchen for easier, more consistent mornings.

Chapter 4

Smart Breakfast Shopping

Managing Type 2 Diabetes begins long before breakfast is served. It starts in the grocery store, where choices made in a short amount of time can either support or complicate your mornings. Shopping with intention helps remove stress from daily decision-making and sets the foundation for balanced, reliable breakfasts.

Smart breakfast shopping is not about finding specialty products or expensive alternatives. It is about knowing what to look for, what to limit, and how to choose foods that support steady blood sugar levels.

Navigating the Breakfast Aisles with Confidence

Many breakfast foods are marketed as healthy, yet contain added sugars, refined grains, or misleading labels. Flavored yogurts, breakfast bars, and packaged cereals often appear convenient but may lead to unexpected blood sugar spikes.

Instead of focusing on marketing claims, pay attention to ingredient lists and nutrition information. Foods with shorter ingredient lists and recognizable ingredients are often better choices. Look for products that contain protein, fiber, and minimal added sugars.

When shopping for breakfast staples, prioritize whole foods such as eggs, plain yogurt, oats, nuts, seeds, fruits, and vegetables. These ingredients provide flexibility and can be combined in many ways to create balanced meals.

Choosing Carbohydrates Wisely

Carbohydrates do not need to be avoided, but they should be selected carefully. Whole grains such as rolled oats, whole grain bread, and quinoa offer fiber that slows digestion and supports blood sugar stability.

When purchasing packaged items like bread or tortillas, choose options labeled whole grain as the first ingredient. Avoid products where sugar or refined flour appears near the top of the ingredient list.

Fruits are a valuable part of breakfast shopping. Fresh or frozen berries, apples, citrus fruits, and pears provide fiber and nutrients without excessive sugar. Frozen fruits are especially useful for smoothies and can be more affordable and convenient.

Protein and Healthy Fat Essentials

Protein is a cornerstone of a balanced breakfast. Items such as eggs, Greek yogurt, cottage cheese, nut butters, and lean meats help slow digestion and promote fullness.

When choosing yogurt, select plain or unsweetened varieties and add your own fruit or nuts for flavor. For nut butters, look for options with minimal ingredients, ideally just nuts and salt.

Healthy fats, including olive oil, avocados, nuts, and seeds, add satisfaction and help regulate energy levels. Keeping these items on hand makes it easier to create balanced breakfasts without extra effort.

Planning for Convenience

Busy mornings require realistic solutions. Shopping with convenience in mind helps prevent skipped meals or rushed choices.

Pre-washed greens, frozen vegetables, and portioned nuts can save time without sacrificing nutrition. Choosing ingredients that can be prepared quickly or in advance supports consistency, even on demanding mornings.

A simple shopping list focused on breakfast essentials reduces impulse purchases and keeps choices aligned with your goals.

Making Breakfast Shopping Sustainable

Effective breakfast shopping is not about perfection. It is about building habits that are easy to maintain. As you become familiar with reliable staples, shopping becomes faster and more intuitive.

Over time, your kitchen becomes stocked with ingredients that support your mornings, making balanced breakfasts the default rather than the exception.

In the next chapter, we will explore how to organize and prepare your kitchen for easy mornings, including pantry essentials and simple preparation strategies.

Chapter 5

Pantry and Prep for Easy Mornings

Mornings are often busy, and when time is limited, even the best intentions can fall apart. A well-organized pantry and simple preparation strategies make it much easier to stick to balanced breakfasts, especially when managing Type 2 Diabetes.

Preparing your kitchen for success does not require elaborate meal prep routines or hours of advance planning. Small, thoughtful steps can make a meaningful difference.

Stocking a Breakfast-Friendly Pantry

A reliable breakfast pantry is built around versatility. Ingredients that can be used in multiple ways help reduce decision fatigue and make breakfast preparation faster.

Whole grains such as rolled oats, quinoa, and whole-grain bread provide a foundation for many meals. These items store well and can be prepared quickly. Nuts and seeds add protein and healthy fats, making them useful for topping bowls, blending into smoothies, or adding to baked recipes.

Healthy fats, including olive oil and nut butters, contribute to satisfaction and help balance carbohydrates. Keeping these staples easily accessible encourages consistent use.

Sweeteners should be chosen carefully. Options such as stevia or small amounts of natural sweeteners can be used intentionally, rather than relying on heavily sweetened packaged foods.

Refrigerated Essentials for Balanced Breakfasts

The refrigerator plays a central role in breakfast preparation. Items such as eggs, plain Greek yogurt, cottage cheese, and fresh produce provide protein and fiber that support blood sugar stability.

Pre-washed greens, chopped vegetables, and washed fruit make it easier to assemble meals quickly. When ingredients are ready to use, it becomes less tempting to skip breakfast or choose less supportive options.

Keeping protein-rich foods at eye level in the refrigerator serves as a simple reminder to include them in morning meals.

Simple Prep Strategies That Save Time

Preparation does not need to be complicated. Cooking grains in advance, portioning nuts, or preparing egg-based dishes ahead of time can significantly reduce morning effort.

Overnight oats, chia puddings, and pre-cooked egg muffins are examples of breakfasts that can be prepared once and enjoyed over several days. These options are especially helpful during busy weeks.

Batch preparation supports consistency without requiring daily cooking. Even preparing just one or two components ahead of time can make mornings feel more manageable.

Reducing Decision Fatigue

One of the most common challenges in diabetes management is decision fatigue. Having too many choices can lead to stress or avoidance.

Creating a short list of reliable breakfast options helps simplify mornings. Rotating a few favorites provides variety without overwhelming the process.

This book is designed to offer many options, but you do not need to use them all at once. Choose what works for your routine and build from there.

Creating a Supportive Morning Environment

A kitchen that supports your goals makes healthy choices easier. When breakfast ingredients are organized and accessible, the path of least resistance becomes the healthier one.

Over time, these small adjustments create a routine that feels natural rather than forced.

In the next chapter, we will focus on portion awareness at breakfast, helping you understand how much is enough without relying on strict rules or constant measurement.

Chapter 6

Portion Awareness at Breakfast

Portion size plays an important role in how breakfast affects blood sugar, energy levels, and overall satisfaction. Even nutritious foods can create challenges when portions are larger than the body needs, especially in the morning when the body is transitioning out of a fasted state.

Portion awareness is not about restriction or constant measuring. It is about learning to recognize what feels balanced and supportive for your body.

Why Portions Matter in the Morning

After waking, the body is particularly responsive to food intake. Large portions of carbohydrates, even high-quality ones, can cause blood sugar levels to rise more quickly than expected. This may lead to fatigue, hunger, or difficulty maintaining focus later in the morning.

Smaller, balanced portions help create a gentler blood sugar response. When carbohydrates are paired with protein and healthy fats, the body processes the meal more slowly, supporting steady energy.

Portion awareness allows you to enjoy a variety of foods while maintaining balance.

Understanding Breakfast Portions Without Measuring Everything

You do not need to weigh food or track numbers at every meal. Visual cues and consistency are often enough.

For grains such as oats or quinoa, moderate portions paired with protein help prevent overconsumption. Fruits are best enjoyed alongside protein or fat, rather than on their own. Protein portions should feel satisfying but not excessive.

Listening to hunger and fullness cues becomes easier when meals are balanced. When breakfast includes protein and fiber, it is easier to stop eating when satisfied.

Common Breakfast Portion Pitfalls

Some breakfast foods appear light but contain more carbohydrates or calories than expected. Granola, fruit smoothies, and baked goods are common examples. Without protein or fiber, these foods may encourage larger portions and faster digestion.

Being mindful of portion size does not mean avoiding these foods. It means adjusting portions and combinations so they support blood sugar balance.

For example, a smaller portion of granola paired with yogurt creates a more balanced meal than granola alone.

Finding What Works for You

Portion needs vary from person to person. Factors such as activity level, body size, and personal response to carbohydrates all play a role.

This book encourages observation rather than perfection. Pay attention to how you feel after breakfast. Steady energy, reduced cravings, and consistent hunger levels are useful indicators that portions are working well for you.

If a meal leaves you hungry too soon or overly full, small adjustments can make a meaningful difference.

Building Confidence Through Routine

Over time, portion awareness becomes intuitive. As you repeat balanced meals, your body adapts, and decision-making becomes easier.

The recipes in this book are designed with portion awareness in mind, offering built-in balance that removes much of the guesswork.

With consistency, breakfast becomes a dependable part of your routine rather than a source of stress.

In the next section, we will transition from foundational guidance to the heart of this book, the breakfast recipes themselves. These recipes put everything you have learned into practice, offering enjoyable, practical meals you can return to again and again.

Bringing It All Together

The foundation you have just explored is not meant to complicate your mornings. It is meant to support them.

Understanding how Type 2 Diabetes interacts with breakfast, learning how to approach carbohydrates without fear, and developing simple habits around shopping, preparation, and portion awareness all serve one purpose. . . to make your mornings easier and more predictable.

Now it is time to put that knowledge into practice.

The breakfast recipes that follow are designed to reflect everything discussed in the previous chapters. Each recipe emphasizes balance, pairing carbohydrates with protein, fiber, and healthy fats to support steady blood sugar levels and sustained energy. All meals are created to be prepared in 30 minutes or less, making them realistic for everyday life.

You do not need to cook every recipe or follow them in order. Choose what fits your schedule, your preferences, and your routine. Some mornings may call for something warm and comforting, while others may require a quick, grab-and-go option. Both are valid and supported here.

As you work through the recipes, allow yourself flexibility. Pay attention to how different meals make you feel, and use that feedback to guide future choices. Over time, patterns will emerge, and confidence will grow.

This section is not about perfection. It is about consistency, enjoyment, and building a breakfast routine that works for you.

Let these recipes support your mornings, nourish your body, and remind you that managing Type 2 Diabetes can be both practical and satisfying.

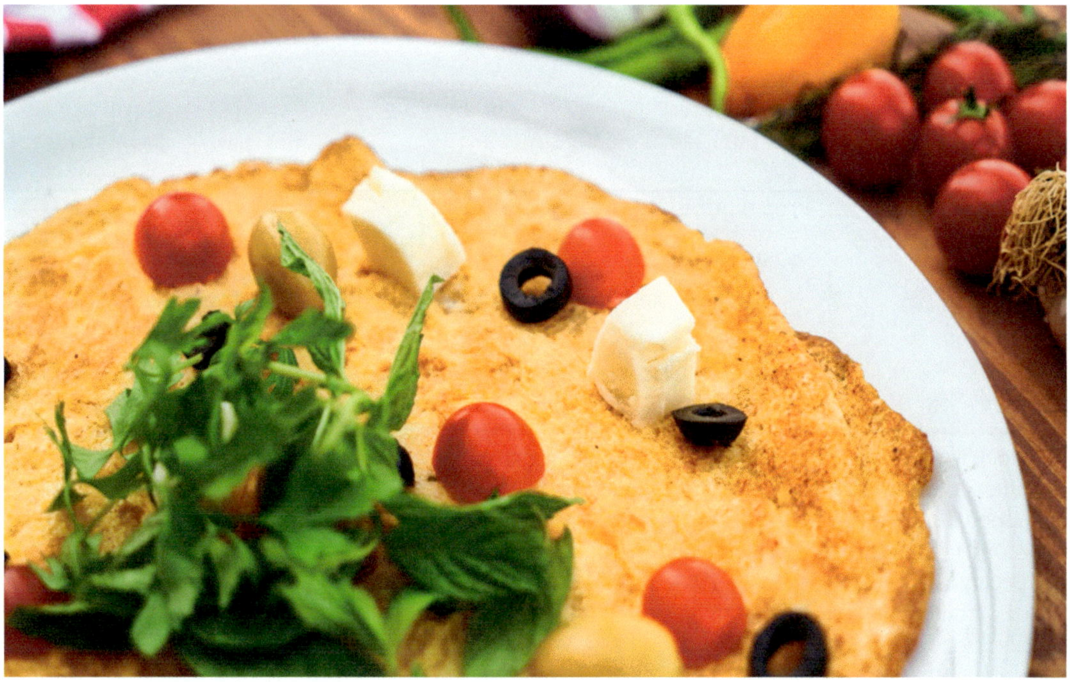

1. Vegetable Omelet

Prep.Time:	Cook Time:	Serving:	Beverage pairing:
5 min	5-7 min	1	Green Tea

Ingredients:

- 2 large eggs
- 1/4 cup diced bell peppers (any color)
- 1/4 cup diced onions
- 1/4 cup diced tomatoes
- 1/4 cup chopped spinach
- 1/4 teaspoon black pepper
- 1/4 teaspoon salt (optional)
- 1 teaspoon olive oil

Preparation:

- In a mixing bowl, beat the eggs until well mixed.
- Add diced bell peppers, onions, tomatoes, chopped spinach, black pepper, and salt (if using) to the eggs. Mix well.
- Heat olive oil in a non-stick skillet over medium heat.
- Pour the egg mixture into the skillet and spread it evenly.
- Cook for 2-3 minutes until the edges start to set.
- Carefully flip the omelette and cook for another 2-3 minutes until cooked through.
- Slide the omelette onto a plate and fold it in half.

Nutrient Facts (per serving):

- Calories: 180
- Carbohydrates: 6g
- Fat: 12g
- Protein: 12g

2. Greek Yogurt Berry Bowl

Prep.Time:	Cook Time:	Serving:	Beverage pairing:
5 min	0 min	1	Herbal Tea

Ingredients:

- 1/2 cup plain Greek yogurt (unsweetened)
- 1/4 cup mixed berries (such as strawberries, blueberries, raspberries)
- 1 tablespoon chopped nuts (almonds, walnuts, or pecans)
- 1 teaspoon chia seeds (optional)
- 1 teaspoon honey or sugar-free sweetener (optional)

Preparation:

1. Spoon Greek yogurt into a bowl.
2. Top with mixed berries, chopped nuts, and chia seeds.
3. Drizzle with honey or sprinkle with a sugar-free sweetener if desired.

Nutrient Facts (per serving):

- Calories: 180
- Carbohydrates: 15g
- Fat: 8g
- Protein: 15g

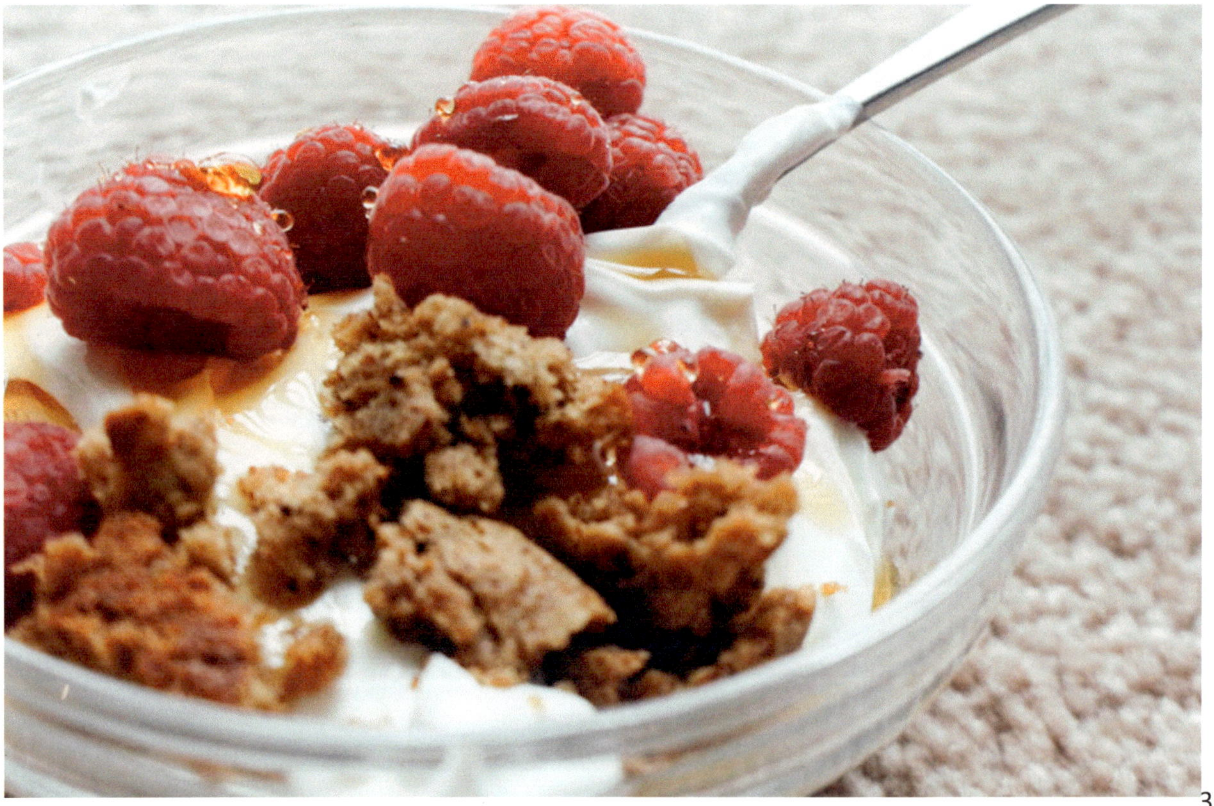

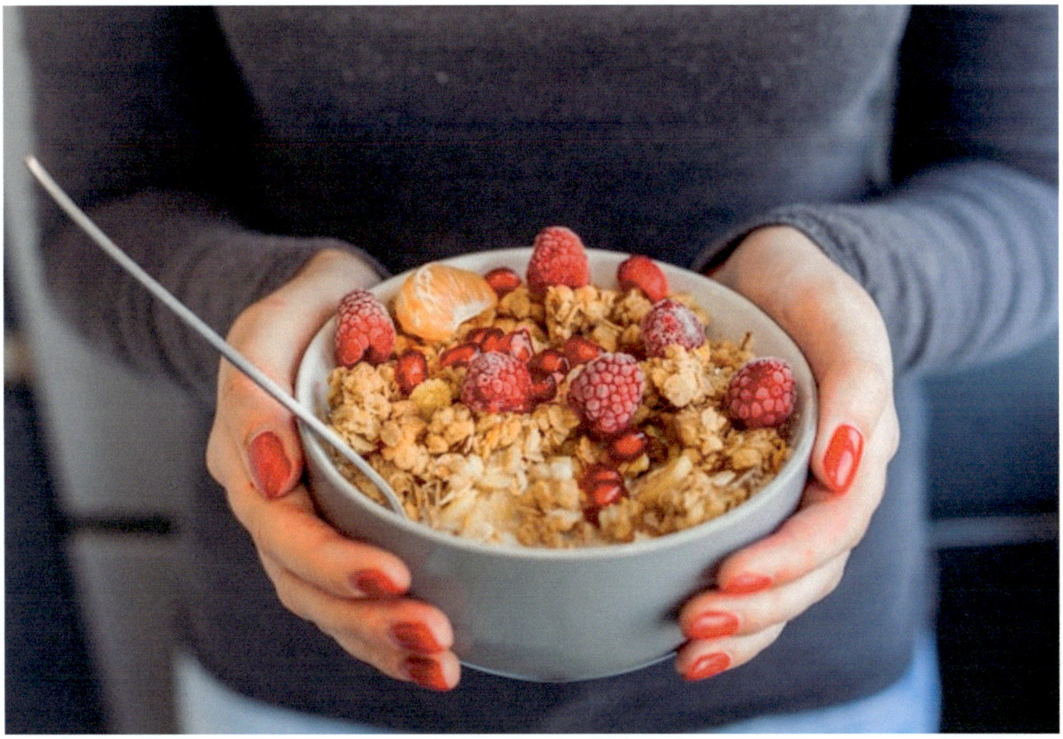

3. Quinoa Breakfast Porridge

Prep.Time: 5 min	**Cook Time:** 20 min	**Serving:** 1	**Beverage pairing:** Black Coffee

Ingredients:

- 1/2 cup quinoa, rinsed
- 1 cup unsweetened almond milk (or any milk of choice)
- 1/4 teaspoon cinnamon
- 1/4 teaspoon vanilla extract
- 1 tablespoon chopped nuts (almonds, walnuts, or pecans)
- 1 tablespoon dried fruits (such as raisins or cranberries)
- 1 sugar-free sweetener (optional)

Preparation:

1. In a saucepan, combine quinoa, almond milk, cinnamon, and vanilla extract.
2. Bring to a boil, then reduce heat to low and simmer for 15-20 minutes, stirring occasionally, until quinoa is cooked and mixture thickens.
3. Stir in chopped nuts and dried fruits.
4. Sweeten with honey or sugar-free sweetener if desired.
5. Serve hot.

Nutrient Facts (per serving):

- Calories: 250
- Carbohydrates: 35g
- Fat: 7g
- Protein: 9g

4. Whole Grain Pancakes with Berries

Prep.Time:	Cook Time:	Serving:	Beverage pairing:
10 min	10 min	1	Herbal Tea

Ingredients:

- 1/2 cup whole wheat flour
- 1 teaspoon baking powder
- 1 tablespoon ground flaxseed
- 1/2 cup unsweetened almond milk (or any milk of choice)
- 1 tablespoon unsweetened applesauce
- 1/2 teaspoon vanilla extract
- 1/4 cup mixed berries (such as strawberries, blueberries, raspberries)

Preparation:

1. In a mixing bowl, whisk together whole wheat flour, baking powder, and ground flaxseed.
2. Add almond milk, applesauce, and vanilla extract. Mix until smooth.
3. Heat a non-stick skillet over medium heat and lightly grease with cooking spray or oil.
4. Pour about 1/4 cup of batter onto the skillet for each pancake.
5. Cook until bubbles form on the surface, then flip and cook until golden brown on both sides.
6. Serve pancakes topped with mixed berries.

Nutrient Facts (per serving):

- Calories: 280
- Carbohydrates: 45g
- Fat: 5g
- Protein: 9g

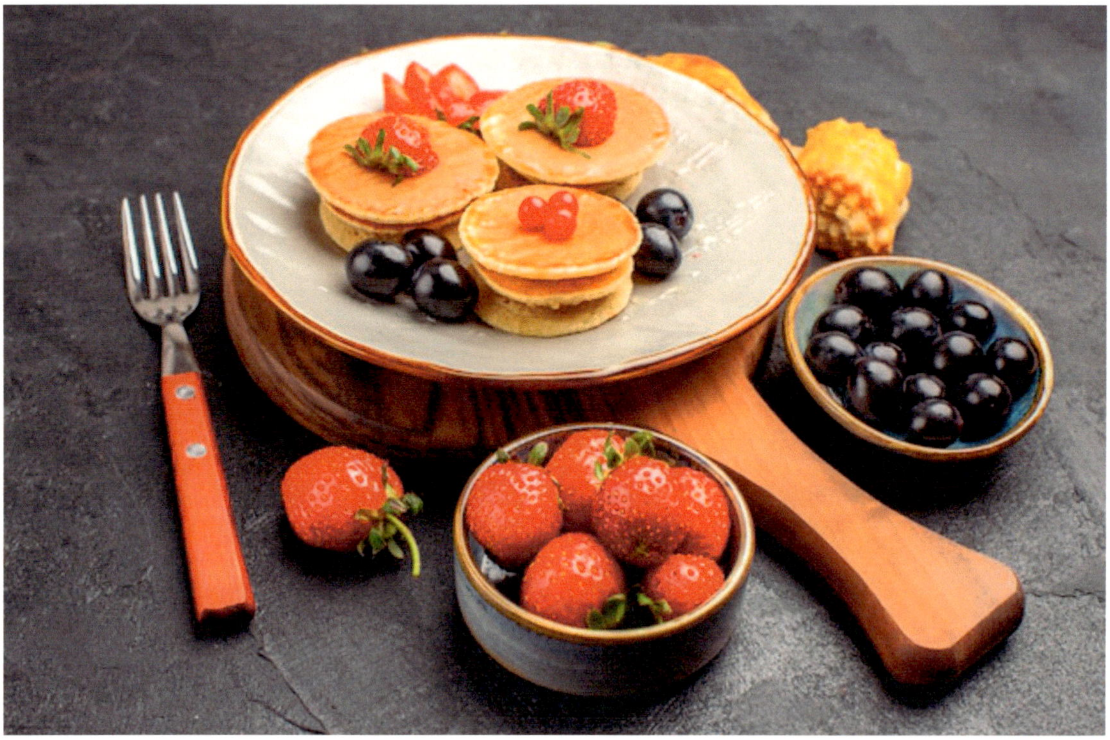

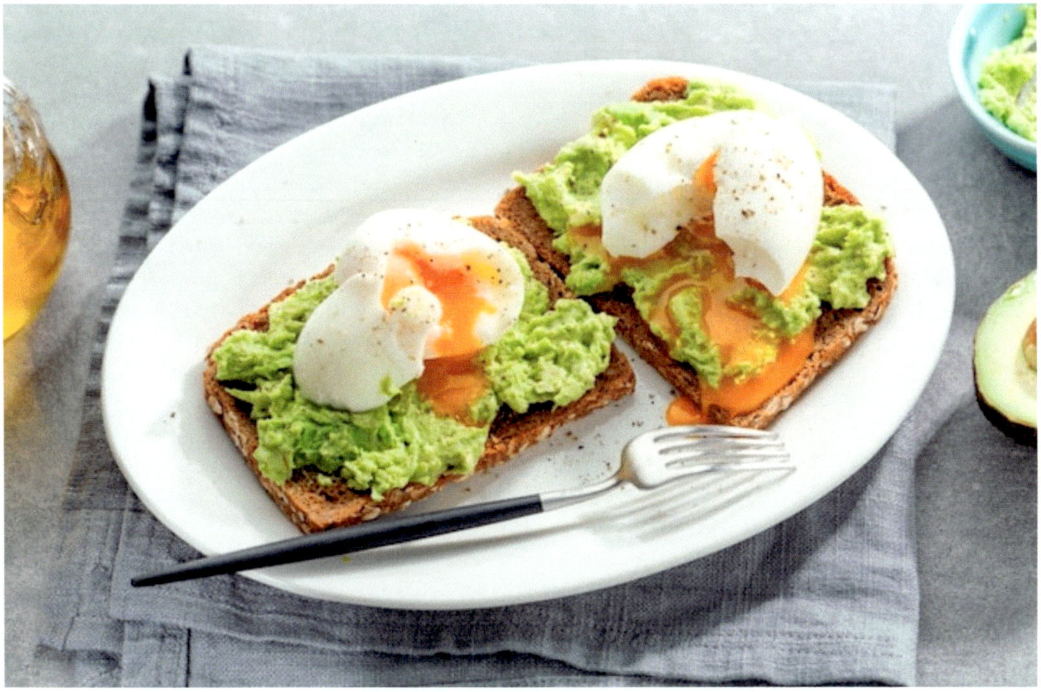

5.Avocado and Poached Egg Toast

Prep.Time: 10 min	**Cook Time:** 5 min	**Serving:** 1	**Beverage pairing:** Black Coffee

Ingredients:

- 1 slice whole grain bread, toasted
- 1/2 ripe avocado, mashed
- 1 poached egg
- Salt and pepper to taste
- Optional toppings: sliced tomatoes, arugula, or hot sauce

Preparation:

1. Toast the whole grain bread until golden brown.
2. Spread mashed avocado evenly on top of the toast.
3. Top with a poached egg.
4. Season with salt and pepper to taste.
5. Add optional toppings if desired.
6. Serve immediately.

Nutrient Facts (per serving):

- Calories: 280
- Carbohydrates: 20g
- Fat: 18g
- Protein: 12g

6. Cottage Cheese Parfait

Prep.Time: 5 min	**Cook Time:** 0 min	**Serving:** 1	**Beverage pairing:** Black Coffee

Ingredients:

- 1/2 cup low-fat cottage cheese
- 1/4 cup mixed berries (such as strawberries, blueberries, raspberries)
- 1 tablespoon chopped nuts (almonds, walnuts, or pecans)
- 1 teaspoon honey or sugar-free sweetener (optional)

Preparation:

1. Spoon cottage cheese into a serving glass or bowl.
2. Layer with mixed berries and chopped nuts.
3. Drizzle with honey or sprinkle with a sugar-free sweetener if desired.

Nutrient Facts (per serving):

- Calories: 200
- Carbohydrates: 15g
- Fat: 8g
- Protein: 18g

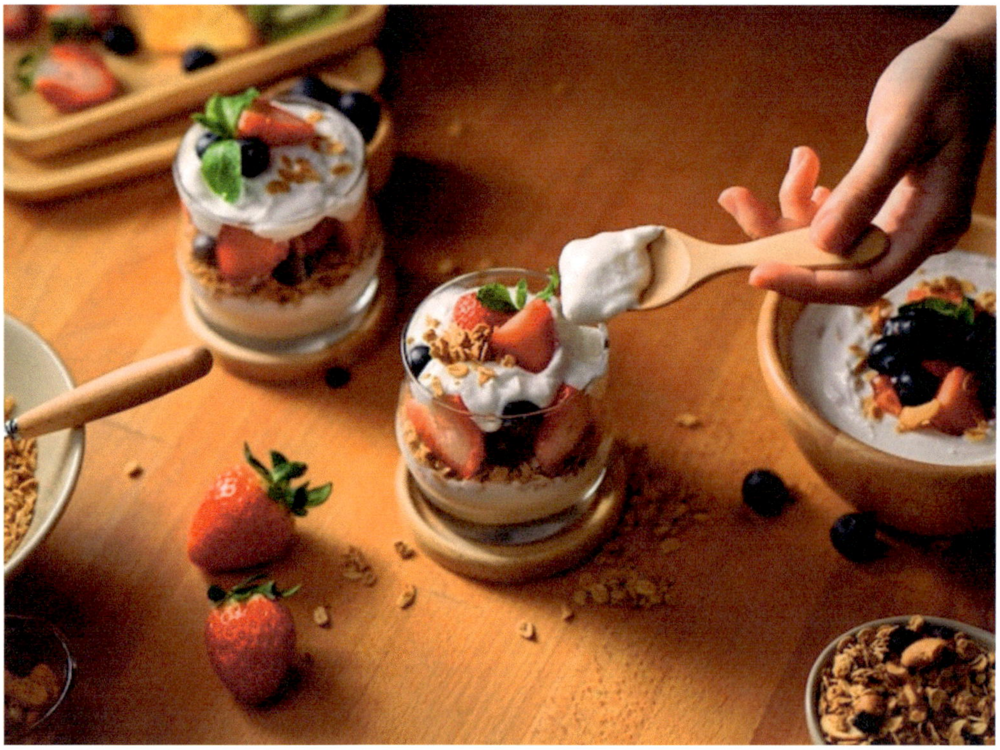

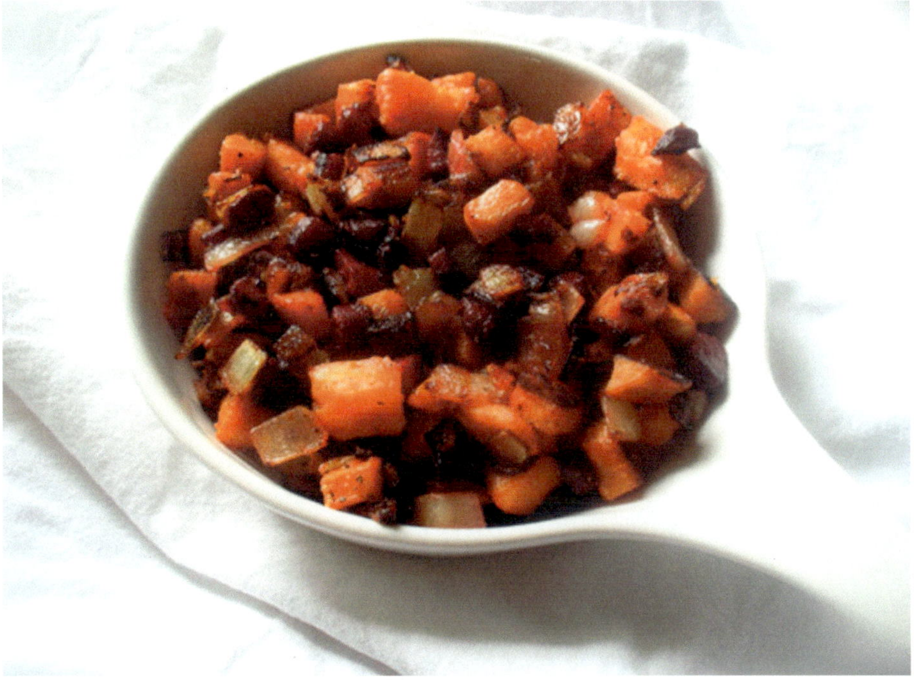

7.Sweet Potato and Turkey Hash

Prep.Time: 10 min	**Cook Time:** 15 min	**Serving:** 1	**Beverage pairing:** Orange Juice

Ingredients:

- 1 small sweet potato, peeled and diced
- 1/4 cup lean ground turkey
- 1/4 cup diced bell peppers (any color)
- 1/4 cup diced onions
- 1/4 teaspoon paprika
- 1/4 teaspoon garlic powder
- Salt and pepper to taste
- 1 teaspoon olive oil

Preparation:

1. Heat olive oil in a skillet over medium heat.
2. Add diced sweet potato and cook until slightly softened, about 5 minutes.
3. Add ground turkey, bell peppers, onions, paprika, garlic powder, salt, and pepper.
4. Cook until turkey is browned and sweet potatoes are cooked through, stirring occasionally, about 8-10 minutes.

Nutrient Facts (per serving):

- Calories: 250
- Carbohydrates: 20g
- Fat: 10g
- Protein: 18g

8.Chia Seed Pudding

Prep.Time: 5 min	**Cook Time:** 0 min	**Serving:** 1	**Beverage pairing:** Black Coffee

Ingredients:

- 2 tablespoons chia seeds
- 1/2 cup unsweetened almond milk
- 1/4 teaspoon vanilla extract
- 1 teaspoon honey or sugar-free sweetener (optional)
- 1/4 cup mixed berries (such as strawberries, blueberries, raspberries)

Preparation:

1. In a bowl, mix chia seeds, almond milk, vanilla extract, and honey (if using). Stir well.
2. Cover the bowl and refrigerate for at least 2 hours or overnight until the mixture thickens.
3. Before serving, stir the pudding and top with mixed berries.

Nutrient Facts (per serving):

- Calories: 150
- Carbohydrates: 15g
- Fat: 8g
- Protein: 5g

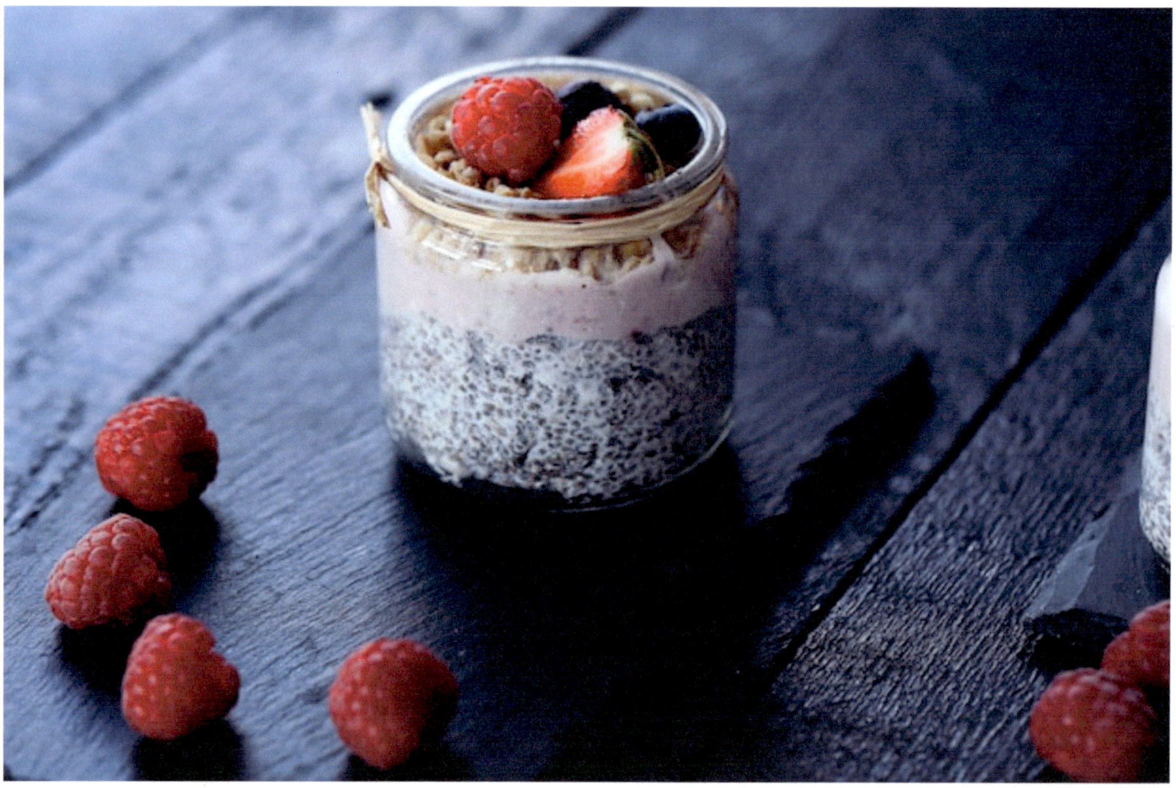

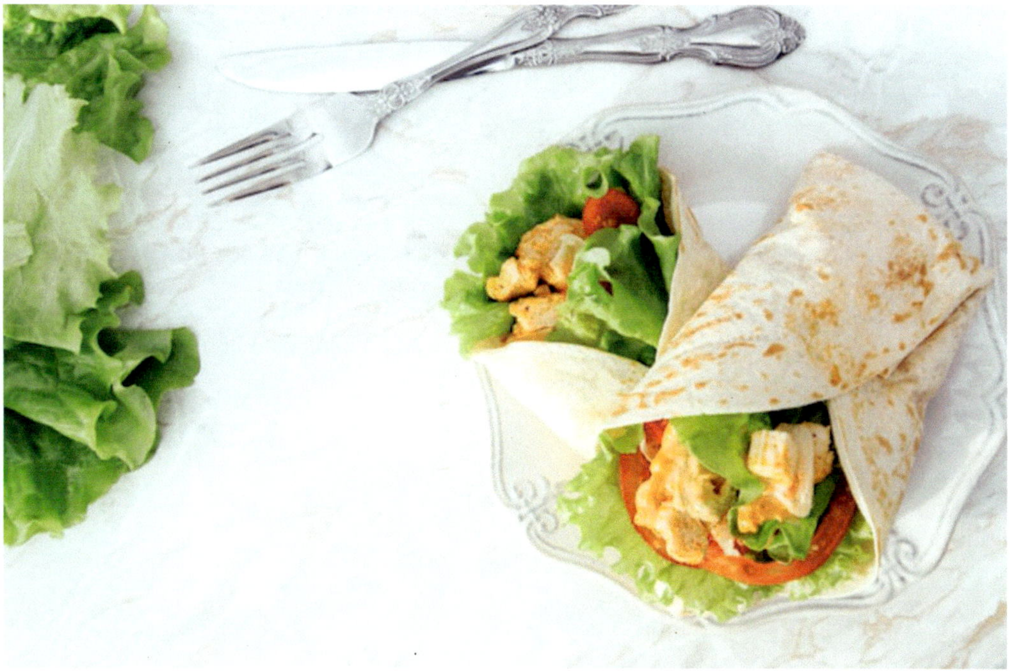

9. Spinach and Feta Breakfast Wrap

Prep.Time: 10 min	**Cook Time:** 5 min	**Serving:** 1	**Beverage pairing:** Orange Juice

Ingredients:

- 1 whole wheat tortilla
- 1/4 cup cooked quinoa
- 1/4 cup baby spinach leaves
- 2 tablespoons crumbled feta cheese
- 1 egg, scrambled
- Salt and pepper to taste
- 1 teaspoon olive oil

Preparation:

1. Heat olive oil in a skillet over medium heat.
2. Place the tortilla on the skillet and warm for about 1 minute on each side.
3. In the center of the tortilla, layer cooked quinoa, baby spinach leaves, scrambled egg, and crumbled feta cheese.
4. Season with salt and pepper to taste.
5. Fold the sides of the tortilla over the filling to create a wrap.

Nutrient Facts (per serving):

- Calories: 320
- Carbohydrates: 30g
- Fat: 15g
- Protein: 15g

10. Almond Butter Banana Smoothie

Prep.Time:	Cook Time:	Serving:	Beverage pairing:
10 min	20-25 min	1	Black Coffee

Ingredients:

- 1 ripe banana
- 2 tablespoons almond butter
- 1/2 cup unsweetened almond milk
- 1/4 teaspoon cinnamon
- 1/4 teaspoon vanilla extract
- Ice cubes (optional)

Preparation:

1. In a blender, combine ripe banana, almond butter, almond milk, cinnamon, and vanilla extract.
2. Blend until smooth.
3. Add ice cubes if desired and blend again until well combined.

Nutrient Facts (per serving):

- Calories: 300
- Carbohydrates: 25g
- Fat: 18g
- Protein: 8g

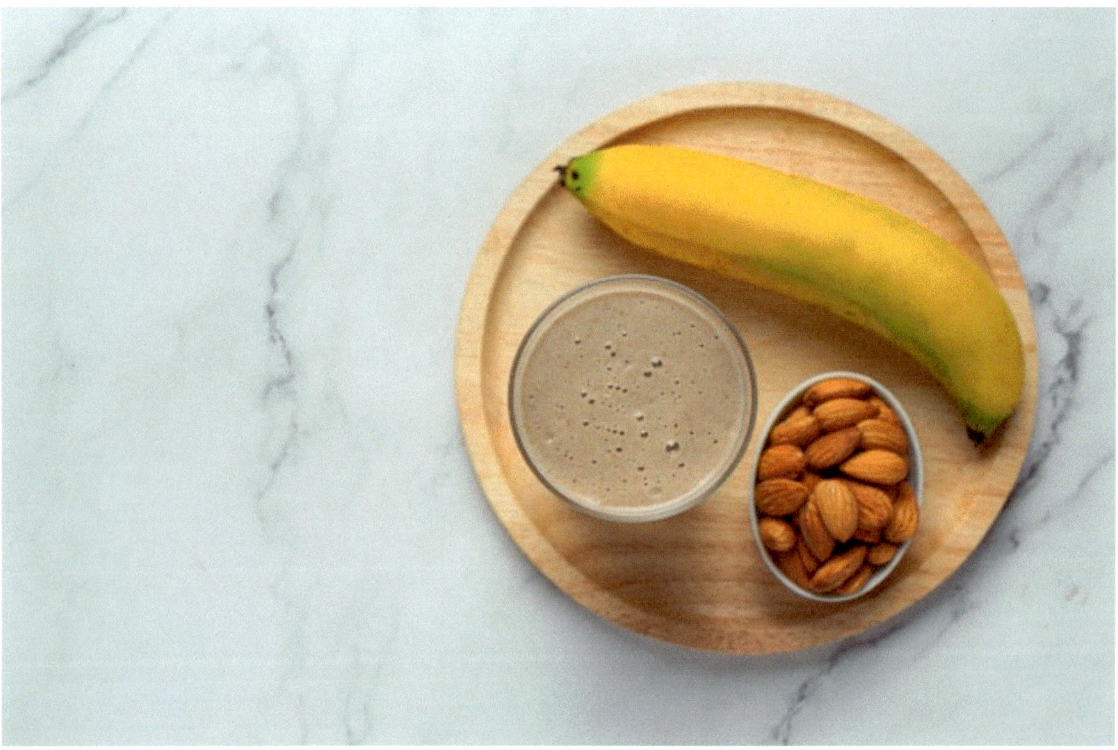

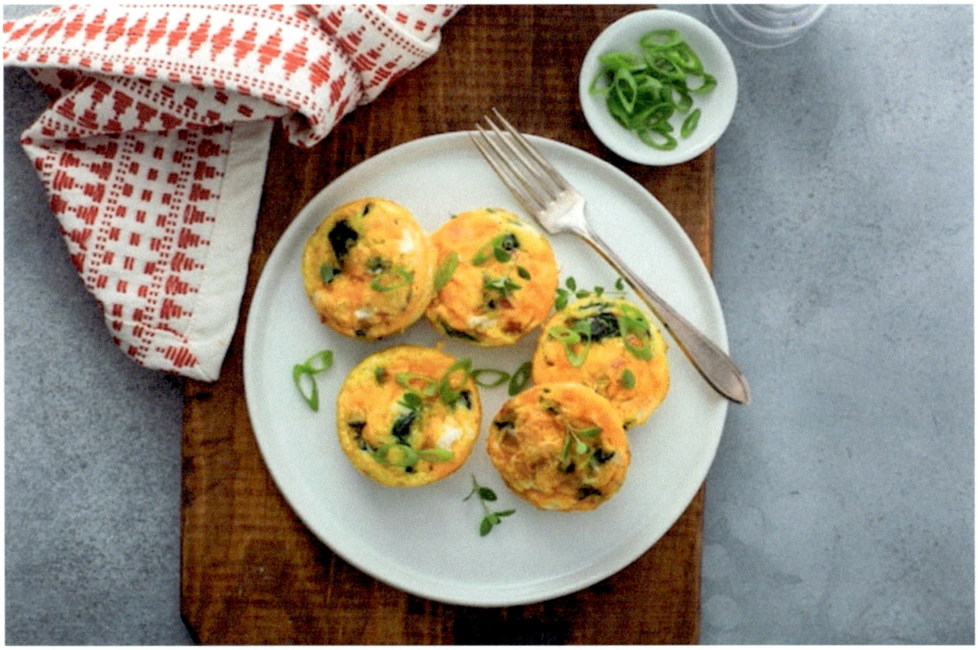

11. Egg Muffins with Veggies

Prep.Time:	Cook Time:	Serving:	Beverage pairing:
10 min	20-25 min	1	Herbal Tea

Ingredients:

- 4 large eggs
- 1/4 cup diced bell peppers (any color)
- 1/4 cup diced onions
- 1/4 cup diced tomatoes
- 1/4 cup chopped spinach
- Salt and pepper to taste
- Cooking spray

Preparation:

1. Preheat the oven to 350°F (175°C). Grease a muffin tin with cooking spray.
2. In a mixing bowl, beat the eggs. Add diced bell peppers, onions, tomatoes, chopped spinach, salt, and pepper. Mix well.
3. Pour the egg mixture evenly into the prepared muffin tin.
4. Bake for 20-25 minutes or until the egg muffins are set and slightly golden on top.
5. Remove from the oven and let them cool slightly before serving.

Nutrient Facts (per serving):

- Calories: 150
- Carbohydrates: 4g
- Fat: 9g
- Protein: 11g

12. Cauliflower and Cheese Breakfast Casserole

Prep.Time: 15 min

Cook Time: 25-30 min

Serving: 4

Beverage pairing: Orange Juice

Ingredients:

- 2 cups cauliflower florets
- 4 eggs
- 1/2 cup shredded cheddar cheese
- 1/4 cup diced onions
- 1/4 cup diced bell peppers (any color)
- Salt and pepper to taste
- Cooking spray

Preparation:

1. Preheat the oven to 375°F (190°C). Grease a baking dish with cooking spray.
2. Steam cauliflower florets until tender, then chop into small pieces.
3. In a mixing bowl, beat the eggs. Add chopped cauliflower, shredded cheddar cheese, diced onions, diced bell peppers, salt, and pepper. Mix well.
4. Pour the mixture into the prepared baking dish.
5. Bake for 25-30 minutes or until the casserole is set and the top is golden brown.
6. Let it cool for a few minutes before slicing and serving.

Nutrient Facts (per serving):

- Calories: 200
- Carbohydrates: 7g
- Fat: 14g
- Protein: 13g

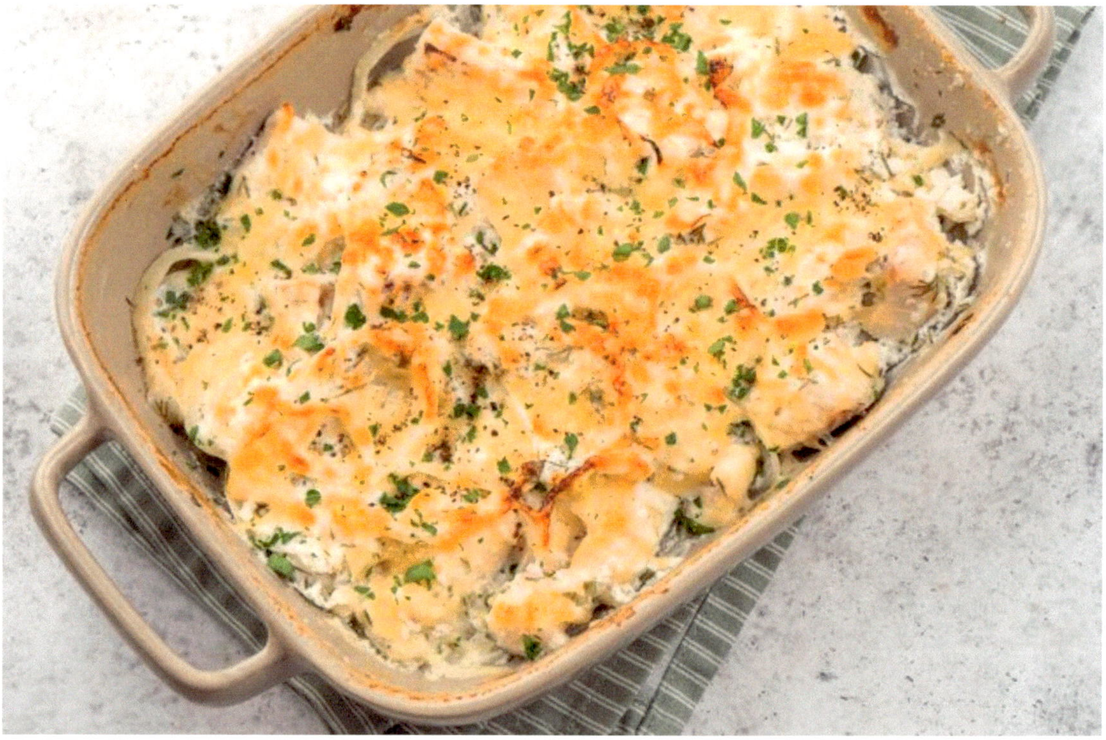

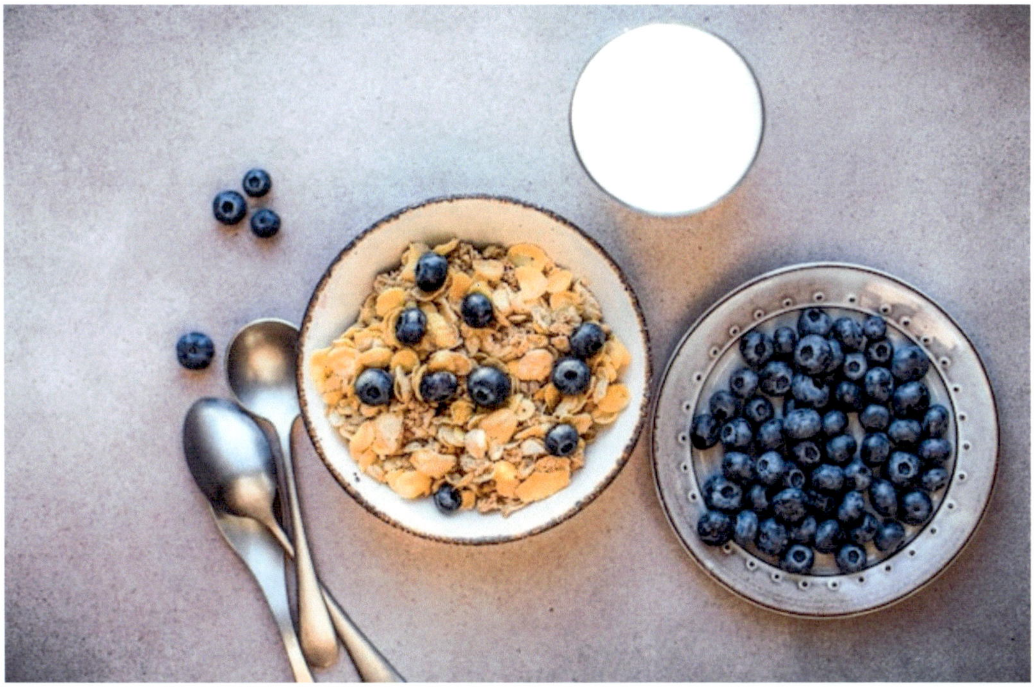

13. Blueberry Almond Overnight Oats

Prep.Time: 5 min

Cook Time: 0 min

Serving: 1

Beverage pairing: Green Tea

Ingredients:

- 1/2 cup rolled oats
- 1/2 cup unsweetened almond milk
- 1/4 cup Greek yogurt (unsweetened)
- 1/4 cup fresh or frozen blueberries
- 1 tablespoon almond slices
- 1 teaspoon honey or sugar-free sweetener (optional)

Preparation:

1. In a mason jar or container, combine rolled oats, almond milk, Greek yogurt, blueberries, almond slices, and honey (if using). Stir well to combine.
2. Cover the jar/container and refrigerate overnight or for at least 4 hours.
3. In the morning, give the oats a stir and enjoy cold or warm by heating in the microwave for 1-2 minutes.

Nutrient Facts (per serving):

- Calories: 250
- Carbohydrates: 32g
- Fat: 8g
- Protein: 12g

14. Turkey Sausage and Veggie Skillet

Prep.Time: 10 min

Cook Time: 15 min

Serving: 2

Beverage pairing: Herbal Tea

Ingredients:

- 2 turkey sausage links, sliced
- 1/2 cup diced bell peppers (any color)
- 1/2 cup diced onions
- 1/2 cup diced tomatoes
- 1/2 cup chopped spinach
- 1/2 teaspoon garlic powder
- Salt and pepper to taste
- 1 teaspoon olive oil

Preparation:

1. Heat olive oil in a skillet over medium heat.
2. Add sliced turkey sausage links to the skillet and cook until browned, about 5 minutes.
3. Add diced bell peppers, onions, and garlic powder. Cook until vegetables are tender, about 5 minutes.
4. Stir in diced tomatoes and chopped spinach. Cook for an additional 2-3 minutes until spinach wilts.
5. Season with salt and pepper to taste.
6. Serve hot.

Nutrient Facts (per serving):

- Calories: 250
- Carbohydrates: 10g
- Fat: 15g
- Protein: 18g

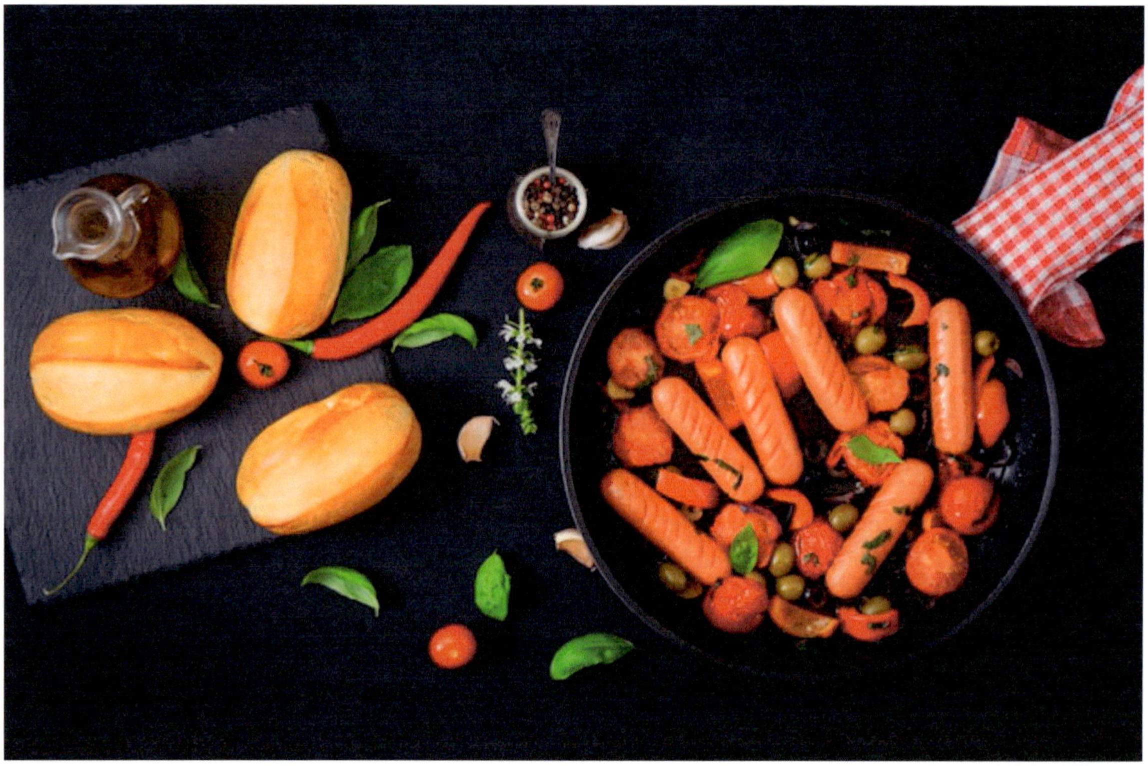

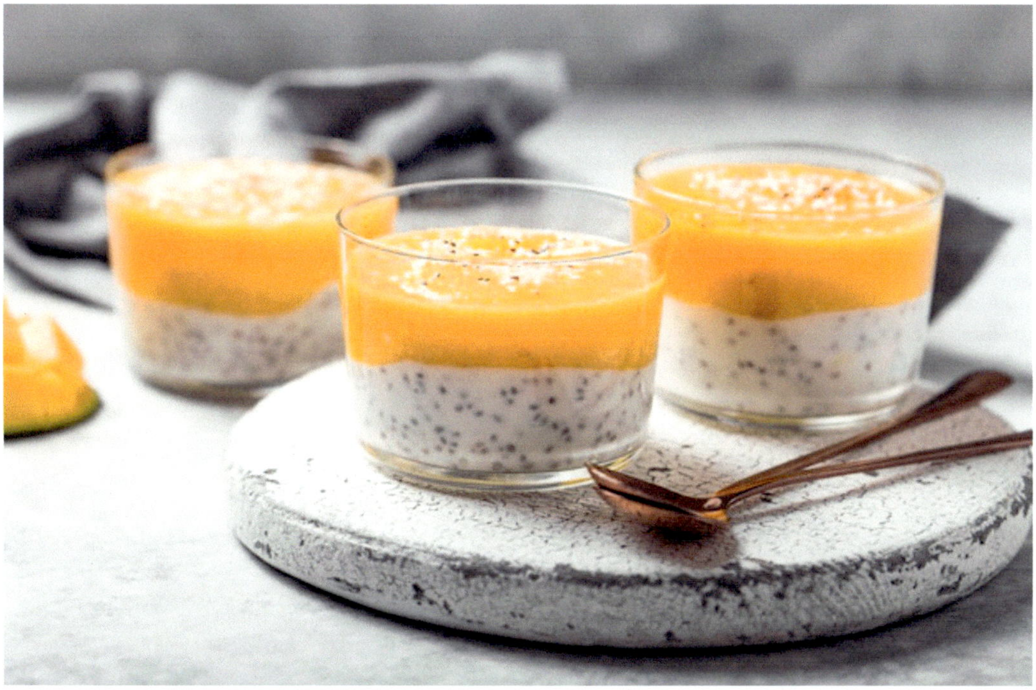

15. Mango Coconut Chia Pudding

Prep.Time:	Cook Time:	Serving:	Beverage pairing:
5 min	0 min	1	Herbal Tea

Ingredients:

- 1/4 cup chia seeds
- 1/2 cup unsweetened coconut milk
- 1/2 cup diced mango
- 1 tablespoon shredded coconut (unsweetened)
- 1 teaspoon honey or sugar-free sweetener (optional)

Preparation:

1. In a bowl, mix chia seeds and coconut milk. Stir well.
2. Cover the bowl and refrigerate for at least 2 hours or overnight until the mixture thickens.
3. Before serving, stir the pudding and top with diced mango and shredded coconut.
4. Drizzle with honey or sprinkle with a sugar-free sweetener if desired.

Nutrient Facts (per serving):

- Calories: 220
- Carbohydrates: 22g
- Fat: 12g
- Protein: 5g

16. Peanut Butter Banana Sandwich

Prep.Time:	Cook Time:	Serving:	Beverage pairing:
5 min	0 min	1	Orange Juice

Ingredients:

- 2 slices whole grain bread
- 2 tablespoons natural peanut butter (unsweetened)
- 1 medium banana, sliced

Preparation:

1. Toast the slices of whole grain bread, if desired.
2. Spread peanut butter evenly on one slice of bread.
3. Arrange sliced bananas on top of the peanut butter.
4. Place the other slice of bread on top to form a sandwich.

Nutrient Facts (per serving):

- Calories: 350
- Carbohydrates: 45g
- Fat: 15g
- Protein: 10g

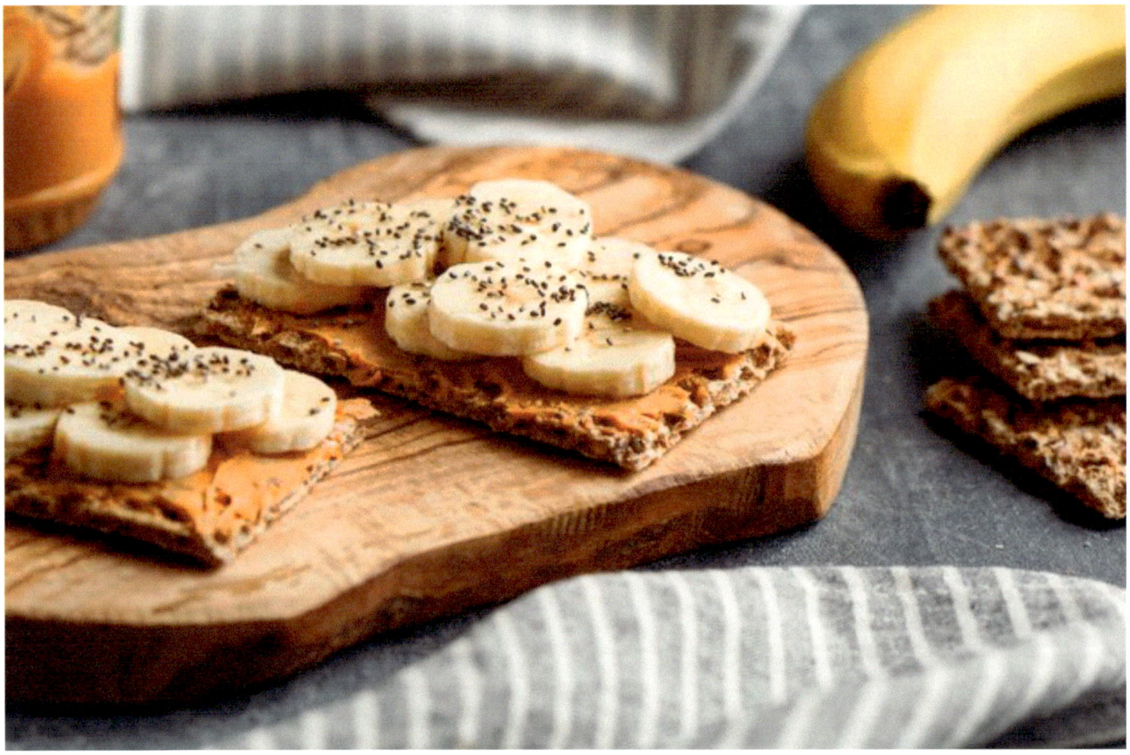

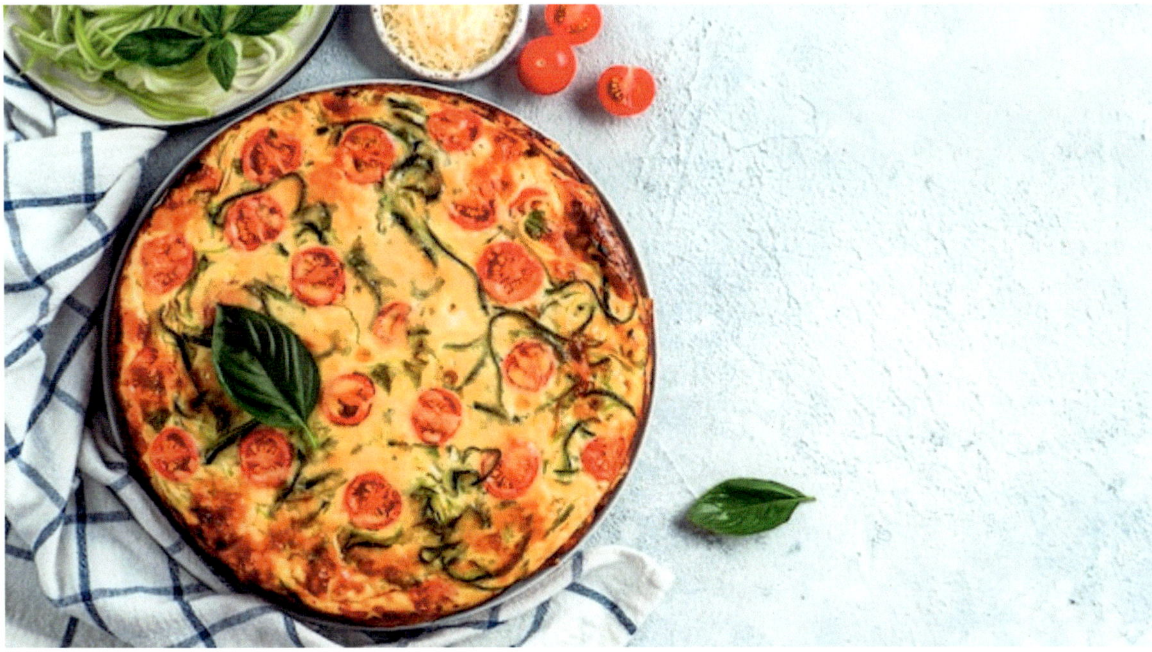

17. Zucchini and Tomato Frittata

Prep.Time:	**Cook Time:**	**Serving:**	**Beverage pairing:**
10 min	10 min	2	Green Tea

Ingredients:

- 4 large eggs
- 1 small zucchini, sliced
- 1/2 cup diced tomatoes
- 1/4 cup diced onions
- 1/4 cup grated Parmesan cheese
- Salt and pepper to taste
- 1 teaspoon olive oil

Preparation:

1. Preheat the broiler in your oven.
2. Heat olive oil in an oven-safe skillet over medium heat.
3. Add sliced zucchini, diced tomatoes, and diced onions to the skillet. Cook until vegetables are tender, about 5 minutes.
4. In a mixing bowl, beat the eggs. Season with salt and pepper, then pour over the vegetables in the skillet.
5. Sprinkle grated Parmesan cheese evenly over the eggs and vegetables.
6. Cook on the stovetop for 3-4 minutes until the edges start to set.
7. Transfer the skillet to the oven and broil for 3-4 minutes until the frittata is set and golden brown on top.
8. Remove from the oven and let it cool slightly before slicing and serving.

Nutrient Facts (per serving):

- Calories: 200
- Carbohydrates: 8g
- Fat: 14g
- Protein: 12g

18. Ricotta and Berry Stuffed French Toast

Prep.Time: 10 min

Cook Time: 10 min

Serving: 2

Beverage pairing: Almond Milk

Ingredients:

- 4 slices whole wheat bread
- 1/2 cup ricotta cheese (low-fat)
- 1/4 cup mixed berries (such as strawberries, blueberries, raspberries)
- 2 large eggs
- 1/4 cup unsweetened almond milk
- 1/2 teaspoon vanilla extract
- 1/4 teaspoon cinnamon
- Cooking spray
- Maple syrup for serving (optional)

Preparation:

1. In a bowl, mix ricotta cheese and mixed berries.
2. Spread the ricotta-berry mixture evenly onto 2 slices of bread. Top with the remaining bread slices to make sandwiches.
3. In another bowl, whisk together eggs, almond milk, vanilla extract, and cinnamon.
4. Dip each sandwich into the egg mixture, ensuring both sides are coated.
5. Heat a non-stick skillet over medium heat and lightly coat with cooking spray.
6. Cook each stuffed French toast sandwich for 3-4 minutes on each side until golden brown and cooked through.
7. Serve hot with maple syrup if desired.

Nutrient Facts (per serving):

- Calories: 300
- Carbohydrates: 30g
- Fat: 10g
- Protein: 18g

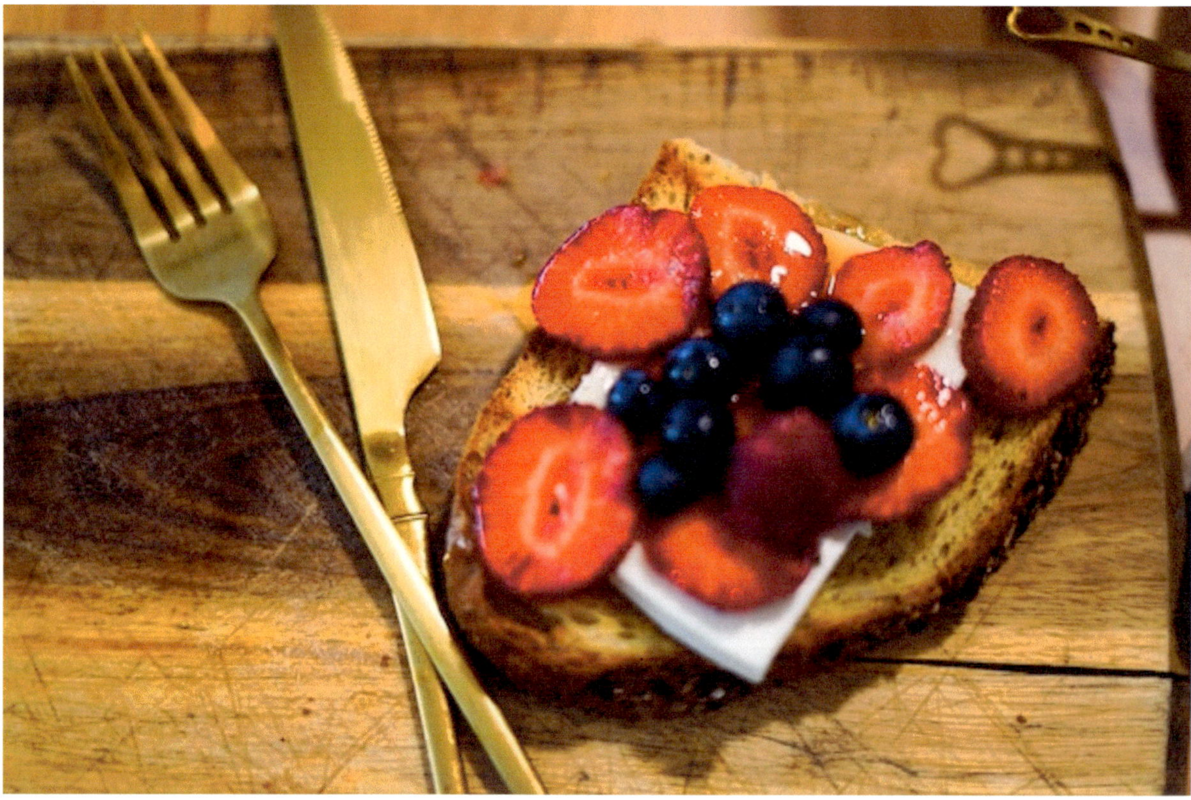

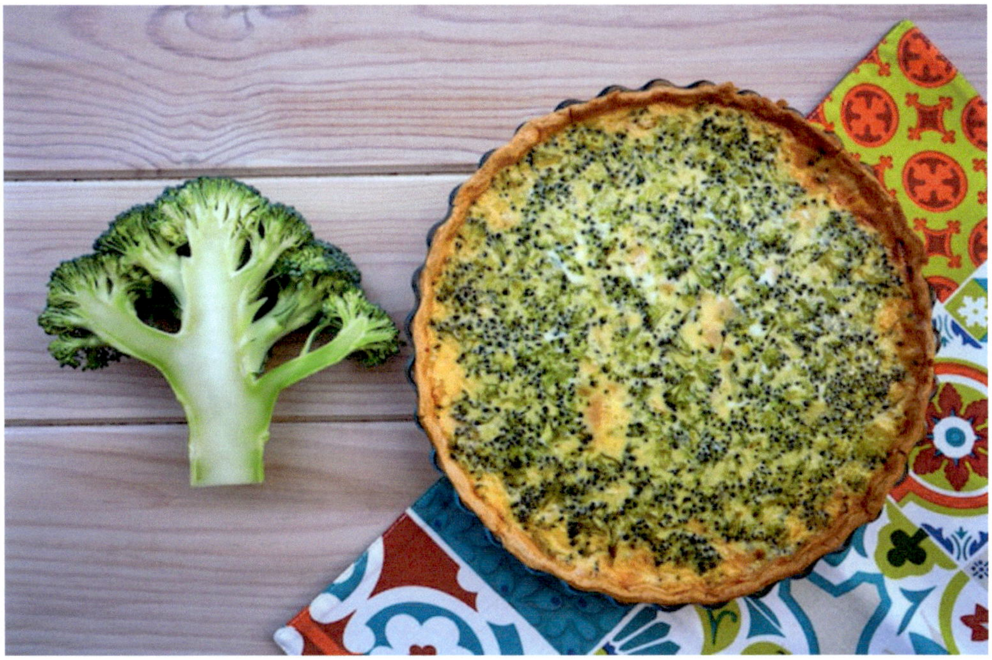

19. Quiche with Spinach and Mushrooms

Prep.Time:	Cook Time:	Serving:	Beverage pairing:
15 min	25-30 min	6	Herbal Tea

Ingredients:

- 1 pre-made whole wheat pie crust (store-bought or homemade)
- 4 large eggs
- 1/2 cup unsweetened almond milk
- 1 cup chopped spinach
- 1 cup sliced mushrooms
- 1/4 cup diced onions
- 1/2 cup shredded mozzarella cheese (part-skim)
- Salt and pepper to taste
- Cooking spray

Preparation:

1. Preheat the oven to 375°F (190°C).
2. In a skillet, sauté chopped spinach, sliced mushrooms, and diced onions until tender.
3. In a mixing bowl, whisk together eggs, almond milk, salt, and pepper.
4. Place the pie crust in a pie dish and spread the sautéed vegetables evenly over the crust.
5. Pour the egg mixture over the vegetables.
6. Sprinkle shredded mozzarella cheese on top.
7. Bake for 25-30 minutes or until the quiche is set and the crust is golden brown.
8. Let it cool for a few minutes before slicing and serving.

Nutrient Facts (per serving):

- Calories: 250
- Carbohydrates: 15g
- Fat: 15g
- Protein: 12g

20. Cherry Almond Breakfast Bowl

Prep.Time:	Cook Time:	Serving:	Beverage pairing:
5 min	0 min	1	Coffee

Ingredients:

- 1/2 cup cooked quinoa
- 1/4 cup unsweetened almond milk
- 1/4 cup dried cherries
- 1 tablespoon almond slices
- 1 tablespoon honey or sugar-free sweetener (optional)

Preparation:

1. In a bowl, combine cooked quinoa and unsweetened almond milk.
2. Top with dried cherries, almond slices, and honey (if using).
3. Stir well to combine.

Nutrient Facts (per serving):

- Calories: 250
- Carbohydrates: 35g
- Fat: 6g
- Protein: 8g

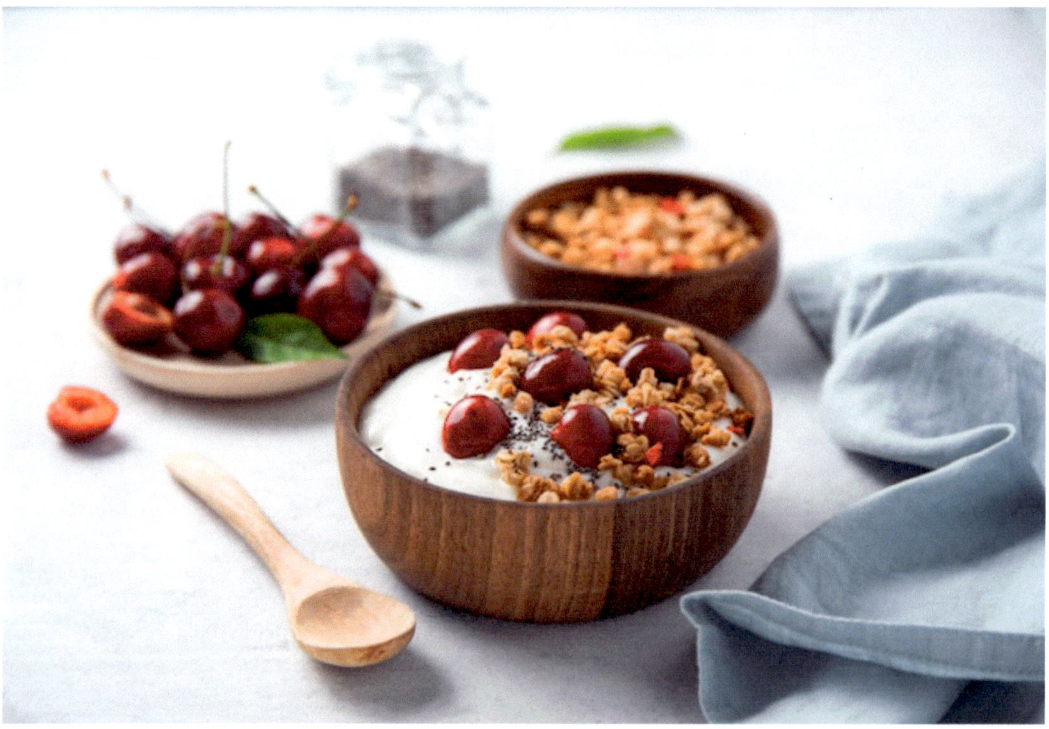

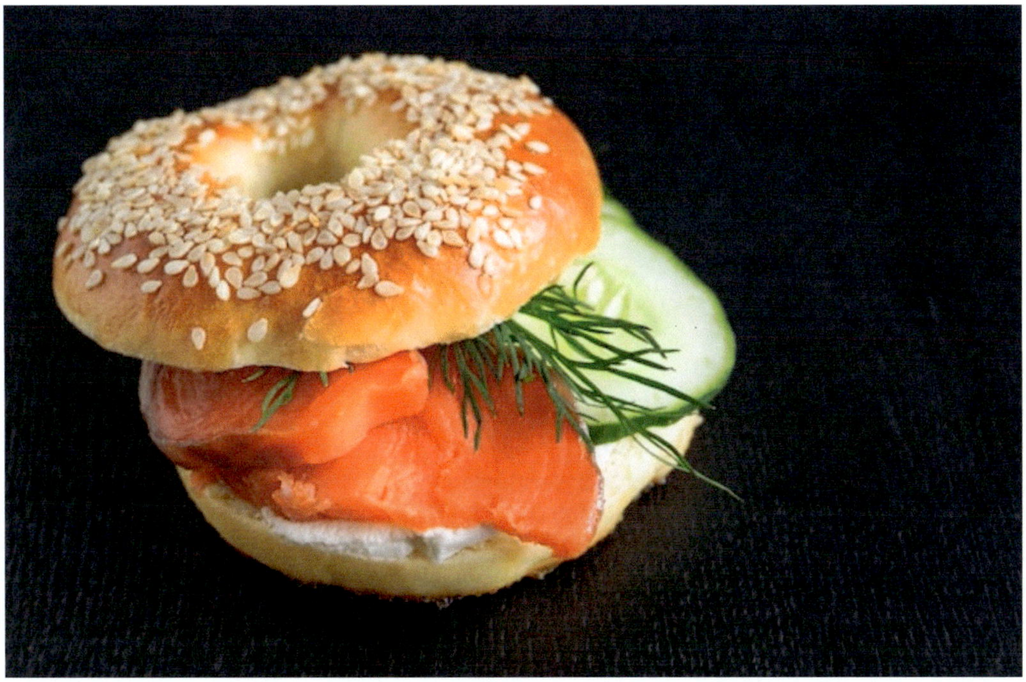

21. Smoked Salmon and Cream Cheese Bagel

Prep.Time:	Cook Time:	Serving:	Beverage pairing:
5 min	0 min	1	Orange Juice

Ingredients:

- 1 whole wheat bagel, sliced and toasted
- 2 tablespoons low-fat cream cheese
- 2 ounces smoked salmon
- 1 tablespoon capers
- 1 tablespoon chopped red onion
- Fresh dill for garnish (optional)

Preparation:

1. Spread cream cheese on each half of the toasted bagel.
2. Top one half with smoked salmon, capers, and chopped red onion.
3. Garnish with fresh dill if desired.
4. Place the other half of the bagel on top to make a sandwich.

Nutrient Facts (per serving):

- Calories: 350
- Carbohydrates: 35g
- Fat: 12g
- Protein: 25g

22. Apple Cinnamon Quinoa Bowl

Prep.Time:	Cook Time:	Serving:	Beverage pairing:
5 min	0 min	1	Herbal Tea

Ingredients:

- 1/2 cup cooked quinoa
- 1/4 cup unsweetened almond milk
- 1/4 cup dried cherries
- 1 tablespoon almond slices
- 1 tablespoon honey or sugar-free sweetener (optional)

Preparation:

1. In a bowl, combine cooked quinoa, diced apple, cinnamon, chopped walnuts, and maple syrup or honey (if using).
2. Stir well to combine.

Nutrient Facts (per serving):

- Calories: 300
- Carbohydrates: 45g
- Fat: 8g
- Protein: 8g

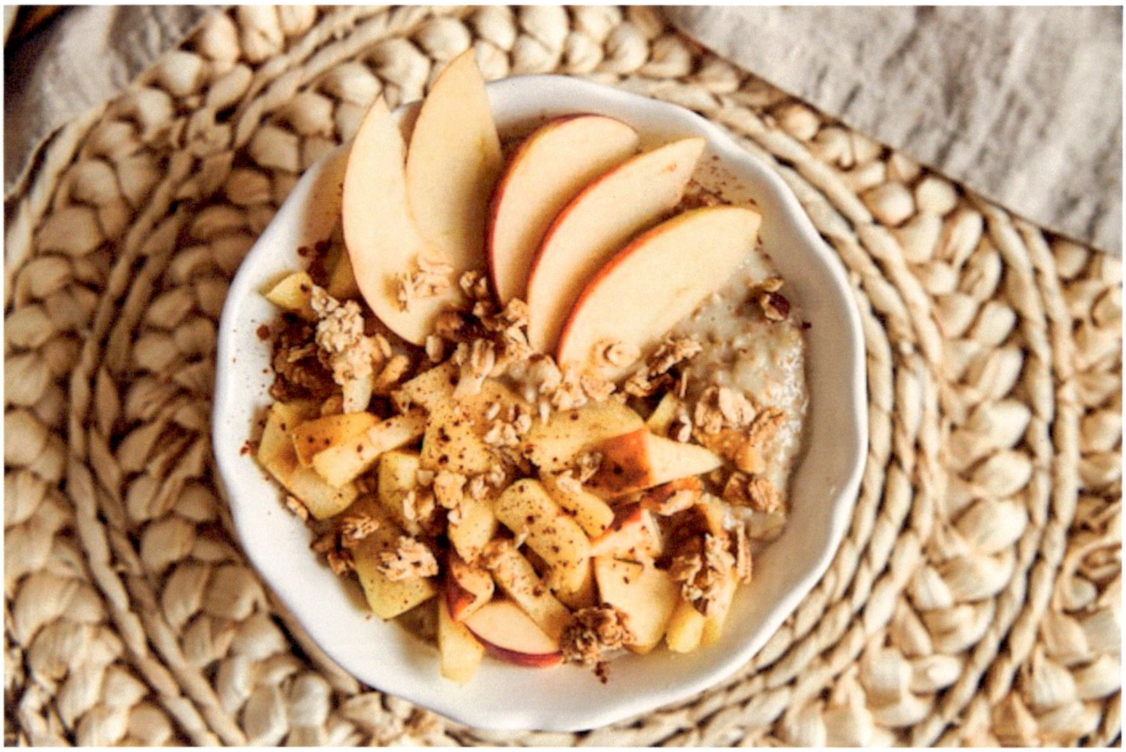

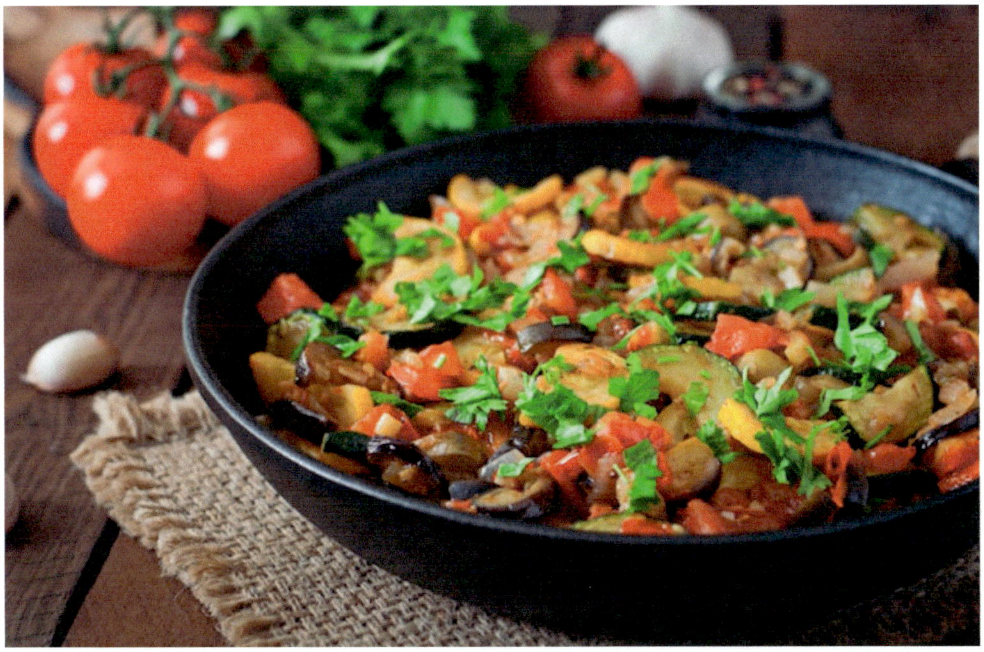

23. Scrambled Tofu with Tomatoes and Spinach

Prep.Time:	Cook Time:	Serving:	Beverage pairing:
10 min	5-7 min	2	Black Coffee

Ingredients:

- 1/2 block (7 oz) firm tofu, crumbled
- 1/2 cup cherry tomatoes, halved
- 1 cup fresh spinach leaves
- 1/4 teaspoon turmeric powder
- Salt and pepper to taste
- 1 teaspoon olive oil

Preparation:

1. Heat olive oil in a skillet over medium heat.
2. Add crumbled tofu to the skillet and cook for 2-3 minutes.
3. Add cherry tomatoes, fresh spinach leaves, turmeric powder, salt, and pepper. Cook for another 2-3 minutes until the spinach wilts and the tomatoes soften.
4. Serve hot.

Nutrient Facts (per serving):

- Calories: 200
- Carbohydrates: 10g
- Fat: 12g
- Protein: 15g

24. Kiwi and Kale Smoothie

Prep.Time:	Cook Time:	Serving:	Beverage pairing:
5 min	0 min	1	Green Tea

Ingredients:

- 1 ripe kiwi, peeled and sliced
- 1 cup chopped kale leaves (stems removed)
- 1/2 frozen banana
- 1/2 cup unsweetened almond milk
- 1/4 cup Greek yogurt (unsweetened)
- 1 tablespoon honey or sugar-free sweetener (optional)
- Ice cubes (optional)

Preparation:

1. Place kiwi slices, chopped kale, frozen banana, almond milk, Greek yogurt, and honey (if using) into a blender.
2. Blend until smooth.
3. Add ice cubes if a colder consistency is desired and blend again until well combined.

Nutrient Facts (per serving):

- Calories: 150
- Carbohydrates: 30g
- Fat: 3g
- Protein: 6g

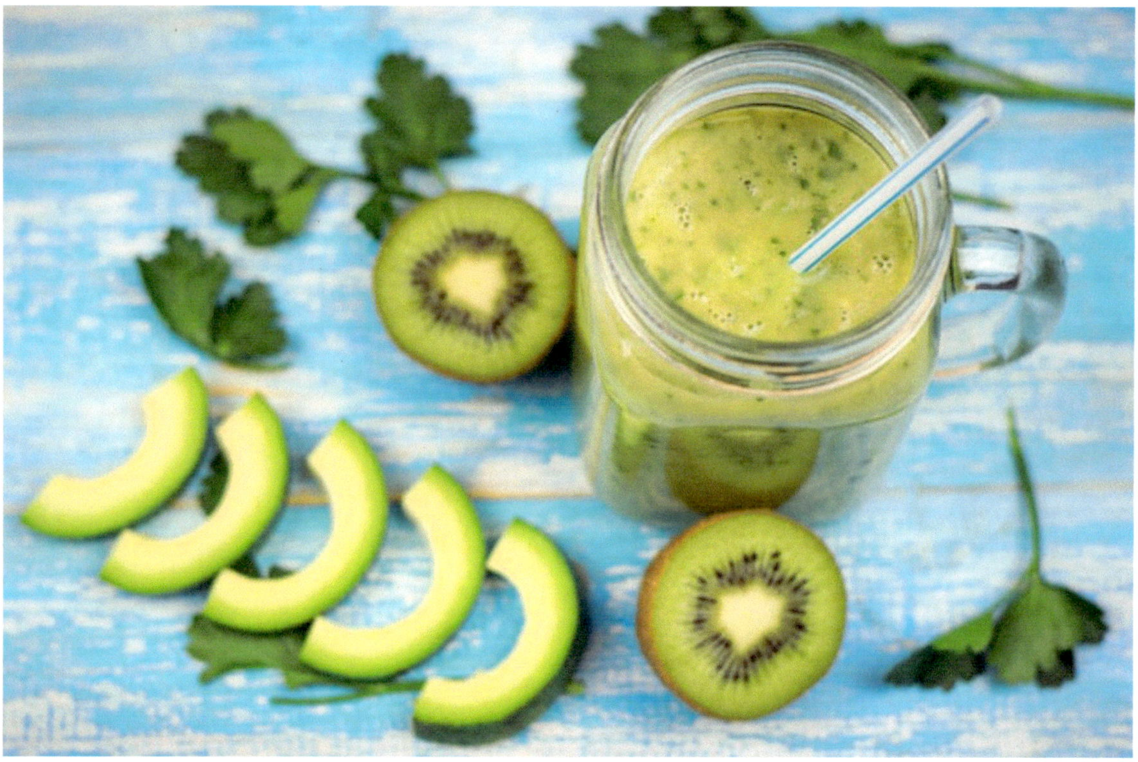

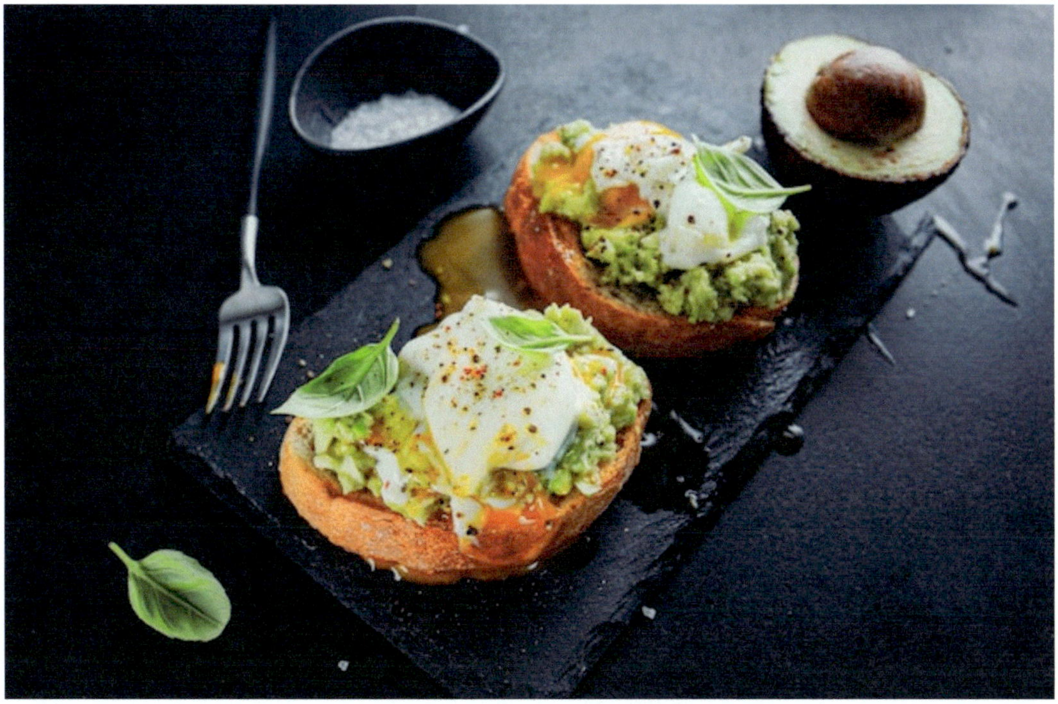

25. Caprese Avocado Toast

Prep.Time: 10 min	**Cook Time:** 0 min	**Serving:** 1	**Beverage pairing:** Grapefruit Juice

Ingredients:

- 2 slices whole wheat bread, toasted
- 1/2 ripe avocado, sliced
- 1 medium tomato, sliced
- 2 slices fresh mozzarella cheese
- Fresh basil leaves
- Balsamic glaze (optional)
- Salt and pepper to taste

Preparation:

1. Spread avocado slices evenly onto the toasted bread slices.
2. Layer tomato slices, fresh mozzarella cheese, and basil leaves on top of the avocado.
3. Drizzle with balsamic glaze if desired.
4. Season with salt and pepper to taste.

Nutrient Facts (per serving):

- Calories: 350
- Carbohydrates: 30g
- Fat: 20g
- Protein: 15g

26. Breakfast Burrito with Black Beans and Salsa

Prep.Time: 10 min

Cook Time: 5 min

Serving: 1

Beverage pairing: Orange Juice

Ingredients:

- 1 whole wheat tortilla
- 2 large eggs, scrambled
- 1/4 cup black beans, drained and rinsed
- 2 tablespoons salsa
- 2 tablespoons shredded cheddar cheese (part-skim)
- Salt and pepper to taste
- Cooking spray

Preparation:

1. Heat a skillet over medium heat and lightly coat with cooking spray.
2. Place the whole wheat tortilla in the skillet and warm for about 1 minute on each side.
3. In the center of the tortilla, layer scrambled eggs, black beans, salsa, and shredded cheddar cheese.
4. Season with salt and pepper to taste.
5. Fold the sides of the tortilla over the filling to create a burrito.

Nutrient Facts (per serving):

- Calories: 350
- Carbohydrates: 30g
- Fat: 15g
- Protein: 20g

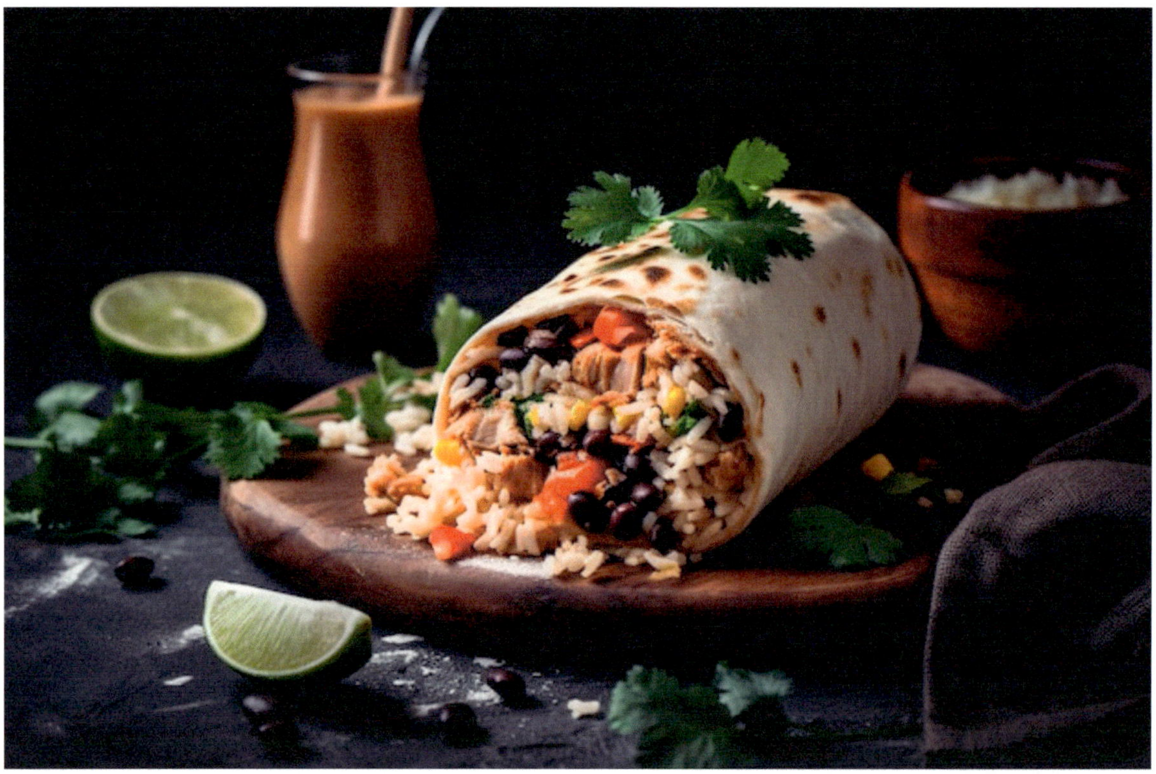

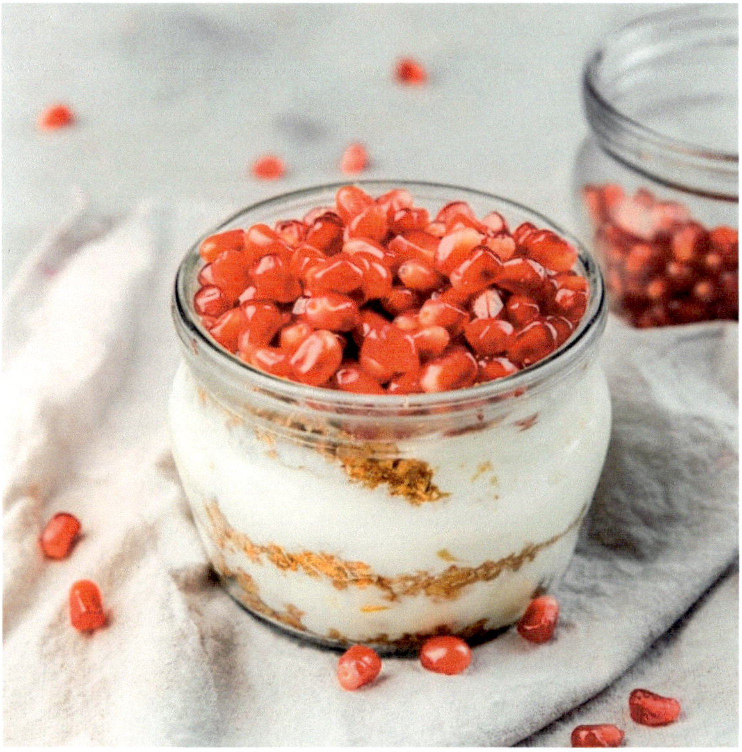

27. Pomegranate and Pistachio Yogurt Parfait

Prep.Time:	Cook Time:	Serving:	Beverage pairing:
5 min	0 min	1	Black Tea

Ingredients:

- 1/2 cup plain Greek yogurt (unsweetened)
- 1/4 cup pomegranate arils
- 2 tablespoons chopped pistachios
- 1 tablespoon honey or sugar-free sweetener (optional)

Preparation:

1. In a glass or bowl, layer plain Greek yogurt, pomegranate arils, and chopped pistachios.
2. Drizzle with honey or sprinkle with a sugar-free sweetener if desired.

Nutrient Facts (per serving):

- Calories: 200
- Carbohydrates: 15g
- Fat: 10g
- Protein: 15g

28. Oat Bran and Berry Muffins

Prep.Time: 10 min	**Cook Time:** 15-18 min	**Serving:** 6	**Beverage pairing:** Herbal Tea

Ingredients:

- 1 cup oat bran
- 1/2 cup whole wheat flour
- 1/4 cup unsweetened applesauce
- 1/4 cup honey or sugar-free sweetener
- 1/4 cup unsweetened almond milk
- 1 large egg
- 1 teaspoon baking powder
- 1/2 teaspoon cinnamon
- 1/2 cup mixed berries (such as blueberries, raspberries)

Preparation:

1. Preheat the oven to 350°F (175°C). Grease a muffin tin or line with muffin liners.
2. In a mixing bowl, combine oat bran, whole wheat flour, applesauce, honey, almond milk, egg, baking powder, and cinnamon. Mix until well combined.
3. Gently fold in mixed berries.
4. Divide the batter evenly into the muffin tin.
5. Bake for 15-18 minutes or until a toothpick inserted into the center comes out clean.
6. Allow the muffins to cool before serving.

Nutrient Facts (per serving):

- Calories: 150
- Carbohydrates: 25g
- Fat: 3g
- Protein: 5g

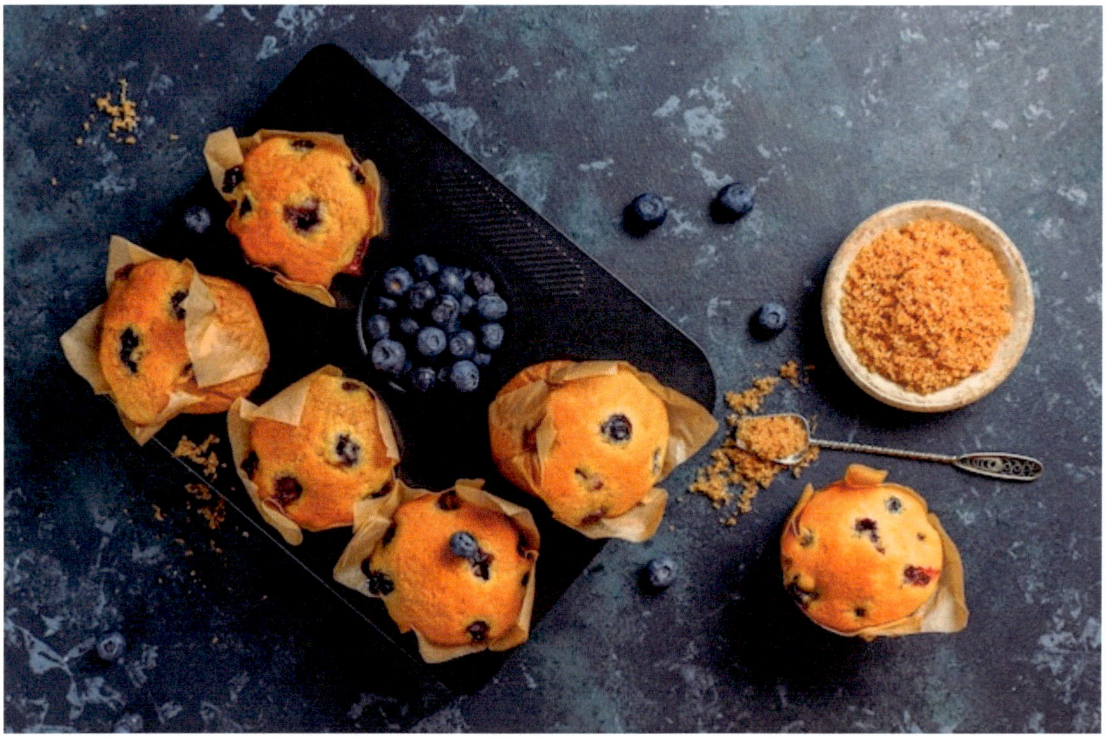

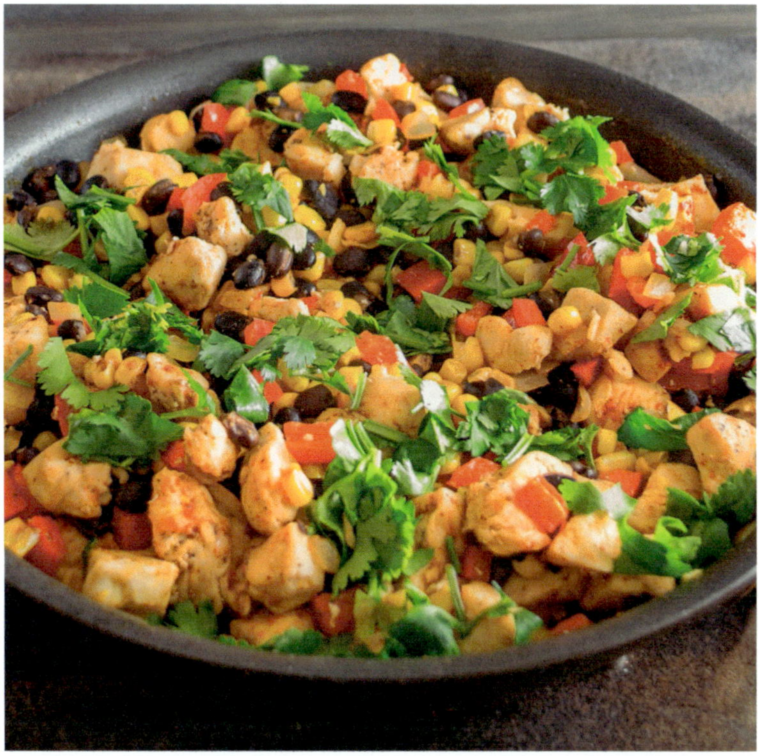

29. Chicken Apple Sausage Breakfast Skillet

Prep.Time: 10 min

Cook Time: 10 min

Serving: 2

Beverage pairing: Black Coffee

Ingredients:

- 2 chicken apple sausages, sliced
- 1/2 cup diced apples
- 1/4 cup diced onions
- 1/4 cup diced bell peppers (any color)
- 2 cups baby spinach leaves
- 1/2 teaspoon paprika
- Salt and pepper to taste
- 1 teaspoon olive oil

Preparation:

1. Heat olive oil in a skillet over medium heat.
2. Add sliced chicken apple sausages and cook until browned, about 3-4 minutes.
3. Add diced apples, onions, and bell peppers to the skillet. Cook until the vegetables are tender, about 5 minutes.
4. Stir in baby spinach leaves and cook until wilted.
5. Season with paprika, salt, and pepper to taste.
6. Serve hot.

Nutrient Facts (per serving):

- Calories: 250
- Carbohydrates: 15g
- Fat: 12g
- Protein: 18g

30. Pear and Walnut Overnight Oats

Prep.Time: 5 min

Cook Time: 0 min

Serving: 1

Beverage pairing: Herbal Tea

Ingredients:

- 1/2 cup rolled oats
- 1/2 cup unsweetened almond milk
- 1/2 ripe pear, diced
- 2 tablespoons chopped walnuts
- 1 tablespoon honey or maple syrup (optional)
- 1/4 teaspoon cinnamon

Preparation:

1. In a jar or container, combine rolled oats, almond milk, diced pear, chopped walnuts, honey or maple syrup (if using), and cinnamon. Stir well.
2. Cover the jar/container and refrigerate overnight or for at least 4 hours.
3. In the morning, give the oats a stir and enjoy cold.

Nutrient Facts (per serving):

- Calories: 300
- Carbohydrates: 40g
- Fat: 10g
- Protein: 8g

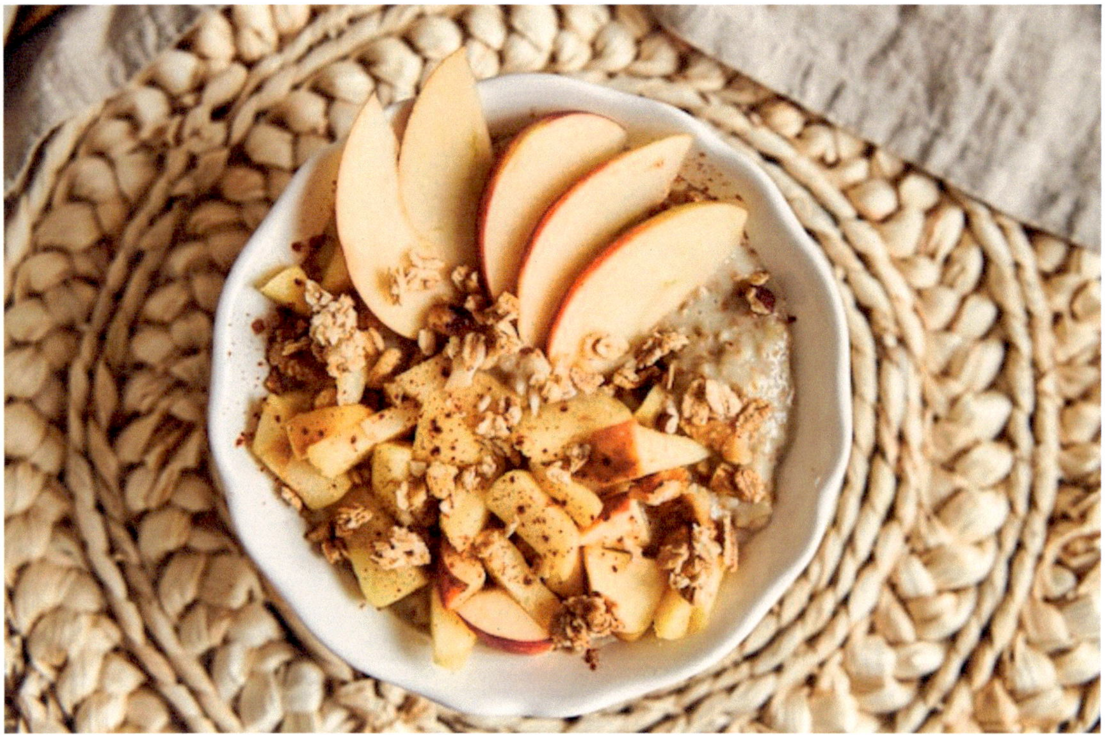

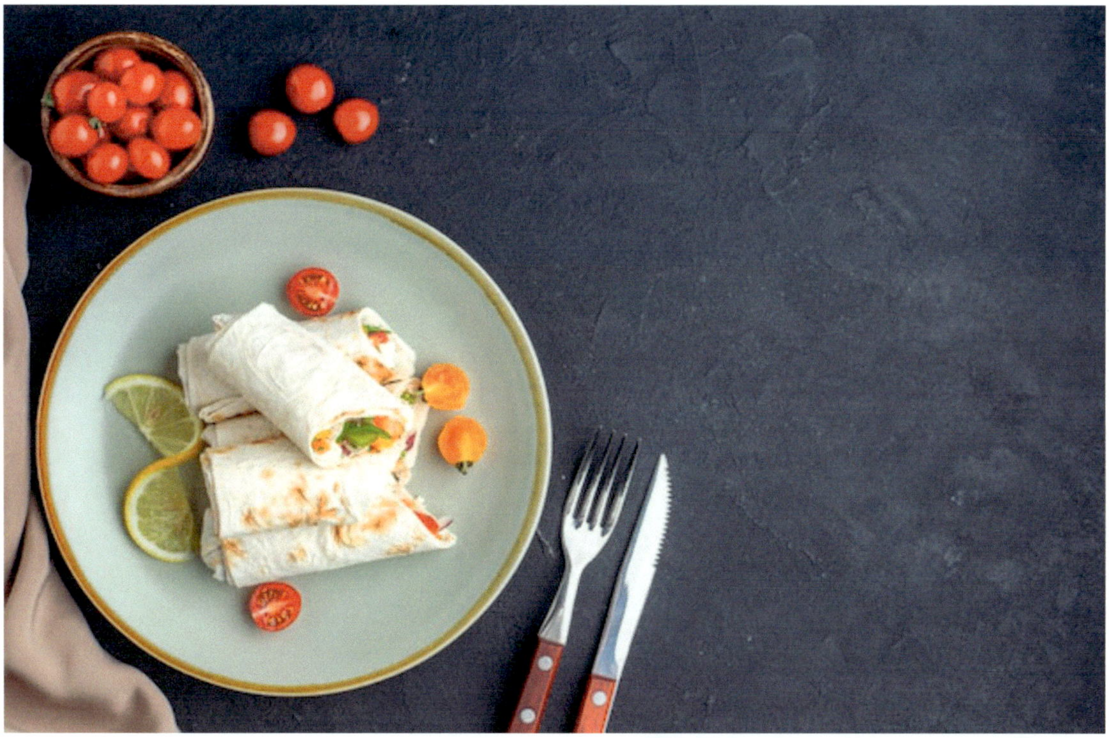

31. Mediterranean Egg White Wrap

Prep.Time:	Cook Time:	Serving:	Beverage pairing:
10 min	5 min	1	Orange Juice

Ingredients:

- 2 large egg whites
- 1 whole wheat tortilla
- 1/4 cup diced tomatoes
- 1/4 cup chopped cucumber
- 2 tablespoons crumbled feta cheese
- 1 tablespoon chopped fresh parsley
- Salt and pepper to taste
- Cooking spray

Preparation:

1. Heat a skillet over medium heat and lightly coat with cooking spray.
2. Pour egg whites into the skillet and cook until set, about 2-3 minutes.
3. Place the cooked egg whites in the center of the whole wheat tortilla.
4. Top with diced tomatoes, chopped cucumber, crumbled feta cheese, chopped fresh parsley, salt, and pepper.
5. Fold the sides of the tortilla over the filling to create a wrap.

Nutrient Facts (per serving):

- Calories: 250
- Carbohydrates: 30g
- Fat: 8g
- Protein: 15g

32. Raspberry Almond Chia Smoothie

Prep.Time:	Cook Time:	Serving:	Beverage pairing:
5 min	0 min	1	Green Tea

Ingredients:

- 1/2 cup frozen raspberries
- 1 tablespoon almond butter
- 1 tablespoon chia seeds
- 1/2 cup unsweetened almond milk
- 1/2 cup Greek yogurt (unsweetened)
- 1 teaspoon honey or sugar-free sweetener (optional)

Preparation:

1. In a blender, combine frozen raspberries, almond butter, chia seeds, almond milk, Greek yogurt, and honey or sugar-free sweetener (if using).
2. Blend until smooth and creamy.
3. Pour into a glass and serve immediately.

Nutrient Facts (per serving):

- Calories: 250
- Carbohydrates: 25g
- Fat: 10g
- Protein: 15g

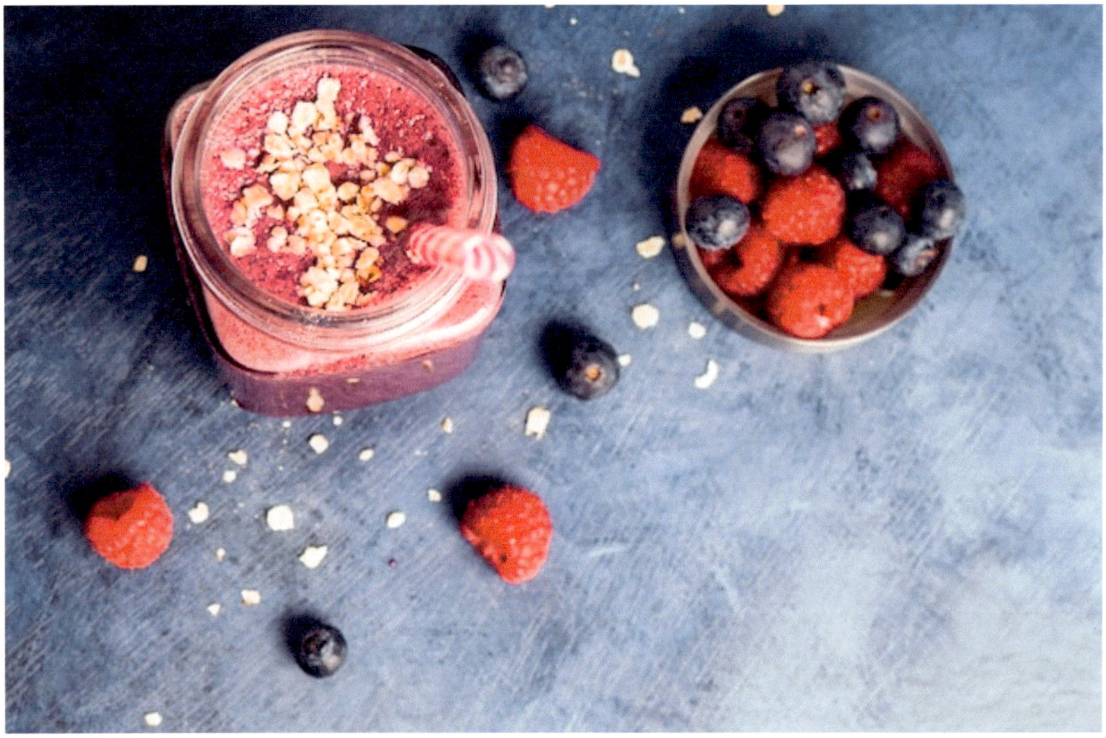

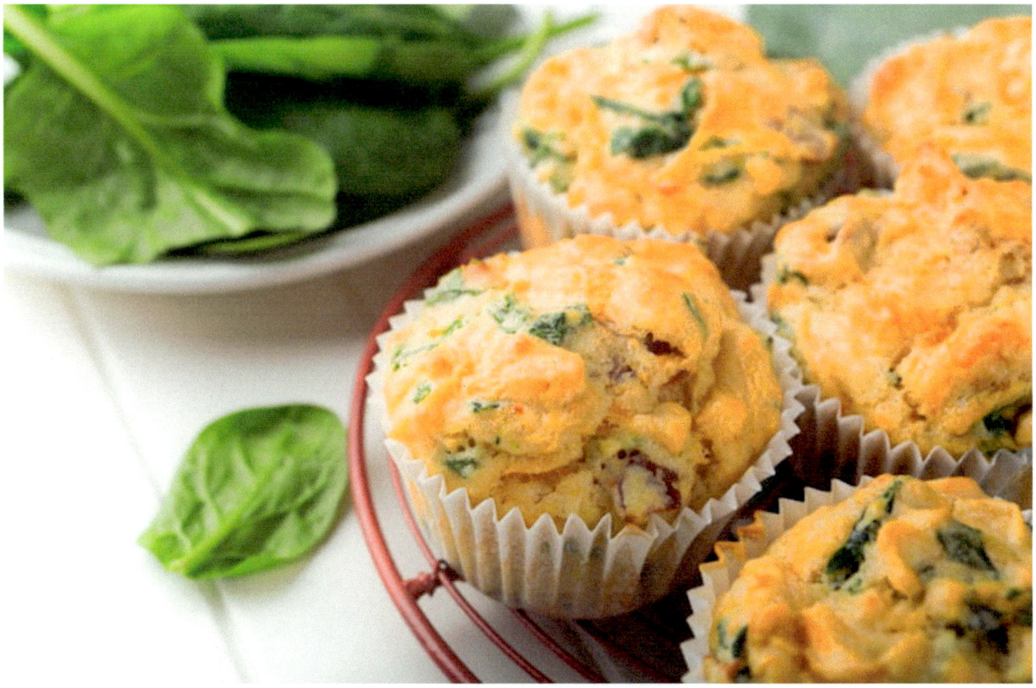

33. Turkey Bacon and Egg Muffin

Prep.Time: 10 min	Cook Time: 0 min	Serving: 1	Beverage pairing: Orange Juice

Ingredients:

- 1 whole wheat English muffin, toasted
- 1 large egg
- 2 slices turkey bacon, cooked
- 1 slice reduced-fat cheddar cheese
- Salt and pepper to taste

Preparation:

1. Cook the egg to your preference (scrambled, fried, or poached).
2. Place the cooked egg on one half of the toasted English muffin.
3. Top with cooked turkey bacon and a slice of reduced-fat cheddar cheese.
4. Season with salt and pepper to taste.
5. Place the other half of the English muffin on top to make a sandwich.

Nutrient Facts (per serving):

- Calories: 300
- Carbohydrates: 30g
- Fat: 12g
- Protein: 18g

34. Cinnamon Raisin French Toast

Prep.Time: 10 min

Cook Time: 10 min

Serving: 1

Beverage pairing: Herbal Tea

Ingredients:

- 2 slices whole wheat bread
- 2 large eggs
- 1/4 cup unsweetened almond milk
- 1/2 teaspoon cinnamon
- 1/4 teaspoon vanilla extract
- 1/4 cup raisins
- Cooking spray
- Maple syrup for serving (optional)

Preparation:

1. In a shallow bowl, whisk together eggs, almond milk, cinnamon, and vanilla extract.
2. Dip each slice of whole wheat bread into the egg mixture, coating both sides evenly.
3. Heat a non-stick skillet over medium heat and lightly coat with cooking spray.
4. Cook each slice of bread for 2-3 minutes on each side until golden brown and cooked through.
5. Sprinkle raisins over the French toast while cooking.
6. Serve hot with maple syrup if desired.

Nutrient Facts (per serving):

- Calories: 300
- Carbohydrates: 35g
- Fat: 10g
- Protein: 15g

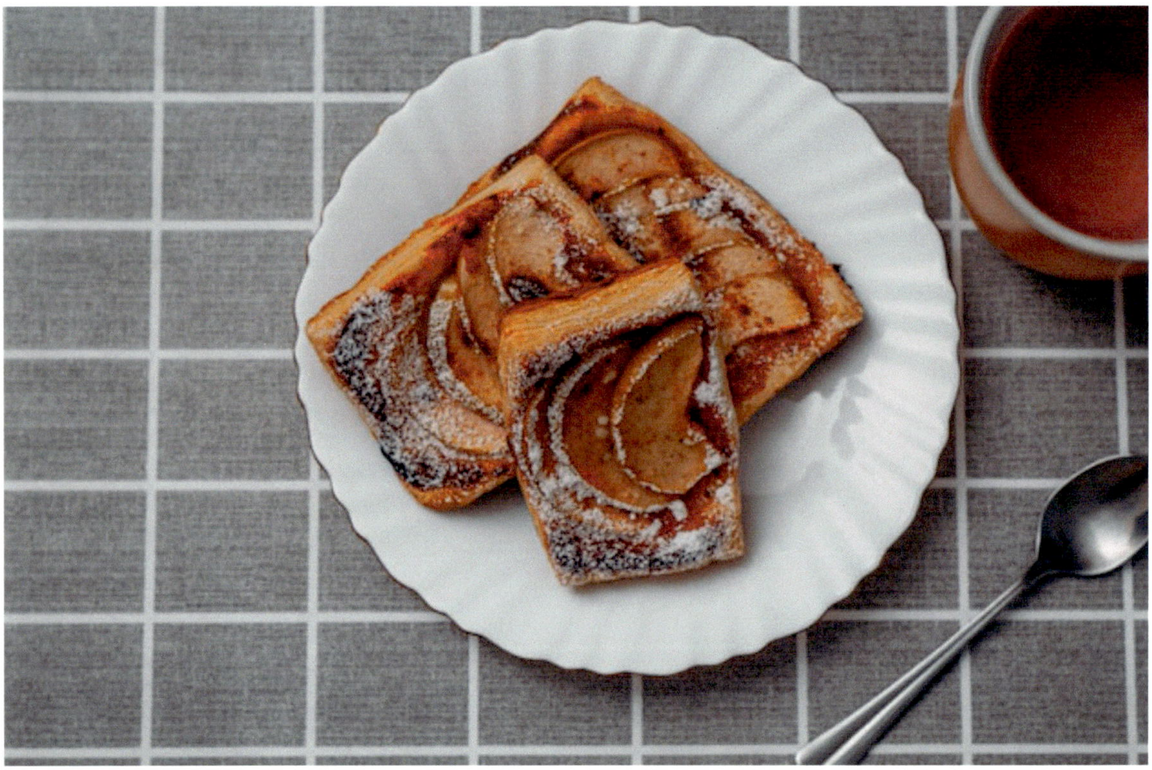

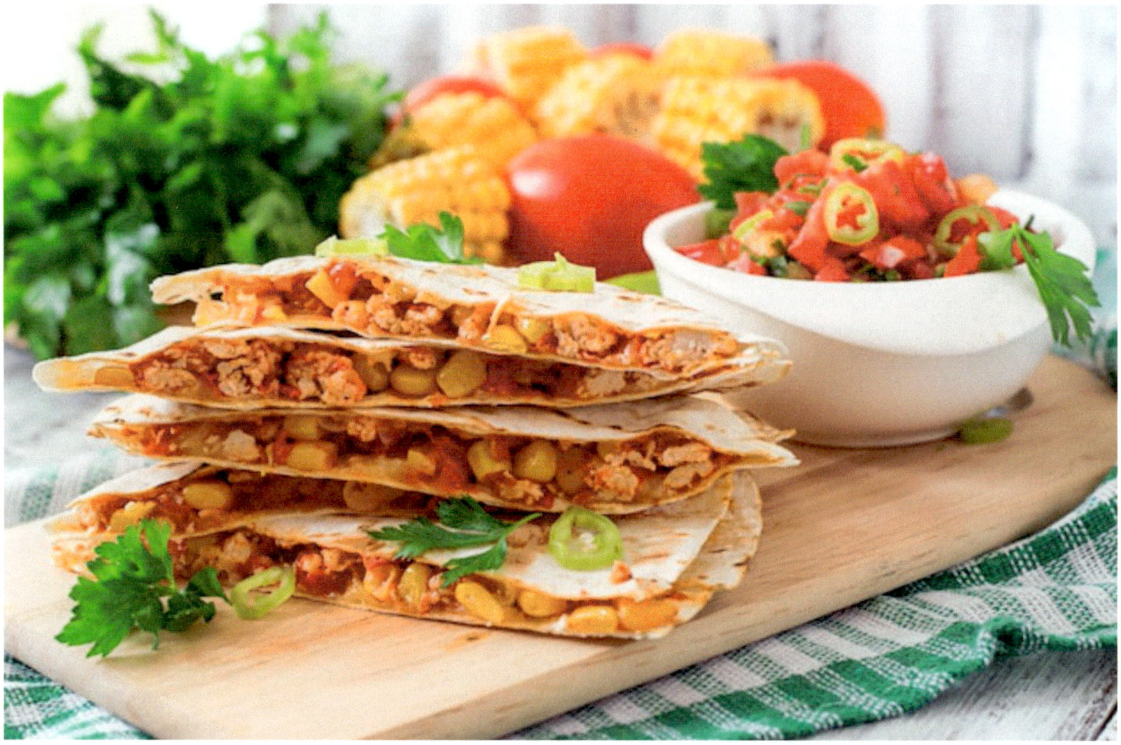

35. Veggie-loaded Breakfast Quesadilla

Prep.Time: 10 min	**Cook Time:** 10 min	**Serving:** 1	**Beverage pairing:** Black Coffee

Ingredients:

- 1 whole wheat tortilla
- 2 large eggs, scrambled
- 1/4 cup diced bell peppers (any color)
- 1/4 cup diced onions
- 1/4 cup diced tomatoes
- 1/4 cup shredded cheddar cheese (part-skim)
- Salt and pepper to taste
- Cooking spray
- Salsa and avocado for serving (optional)

Preparation:

1. Heat a skillet over medium heat and lightly coat with cooking spray.
2. Place the whole wheat tortilla in the skillet and warm for about 1 minute on each side.
3. In a separate pan, scramble the eggs.
4. Spread scrambled eggs evenly over one half of the tortilla.
5. Top with diced bell peppers, onions, tomatoes, and shredded cheddar cheese.
6. Fold the other half of the tortilla over the filling to create a quesadilla.
7. Cook for 2-3 minutes on each side until the cheese is melted and the tortilla is golden brown.
8. Serve hot with salsa and avocado if desired.

Nutrient Facts (per serving):

- Calories: 350
- Carbohydrates: 30g
- Fat: 15g
- Protein: 20g

36. Banana Nut Quinoa Muffins

Prep.Time:	Cook Time:	Serving:	Beverage pairing:
10 min	20-25 min	12	Almond Milk

Ingredients:

- 1 cup cooked quinoa
- 1 ripe banana, mashed
- 1/4 cup chopped walnuts
- 1/4 cup honey or maple syrup
- 2 eggs
- 1/4 cup unsweetened almond milk
- 1 teaspoon vanilla extract
- 1 teaspoon baking powder
- 1/2 teaspoon cinnamon
- Pinch of salt

Preparation:

1. Preheat the oven to 350°F (175°C) and line a muffin tin with liners or grease it lightly.
2. In a large bowl, mix together mashed banana, honey or maple syrup, eggs, almond milk, and vanilla extract until well combined.
3. In another bowl, combine cooked quinoa, chopped walnuts, baking powder, cinnamon, and salt.
4. Gradually add the dry ingredients to the wet ingredients, stirring until just combined.
5. Spoon the batter into the muffin tin, filling each cup about 3/4 full.
6. Bake for 20-25 minutes or until a toothpick inserted into the center of a muffin comes out clean.
7. Allow the muffins to cool in the tin for 5 minutes before transferring to a wire rack to cool completely.

Nutrient Facts (per serving):

- Calories: 150
- Carbohydrates: 20g
- Fat: 6g
- Protein: 5g

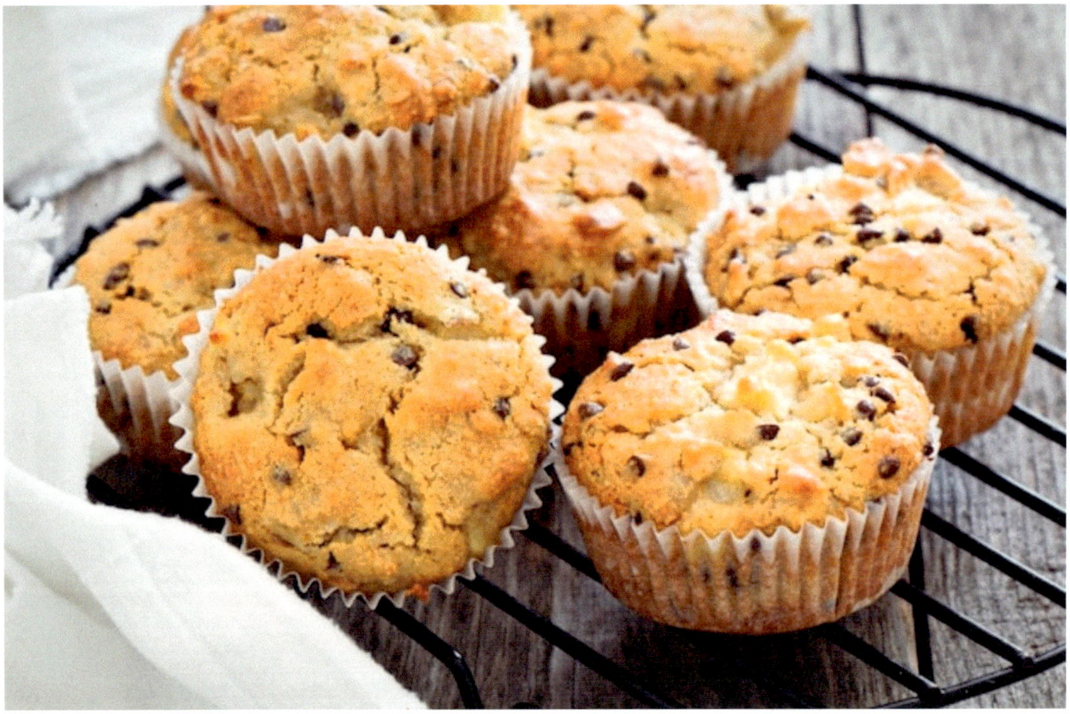

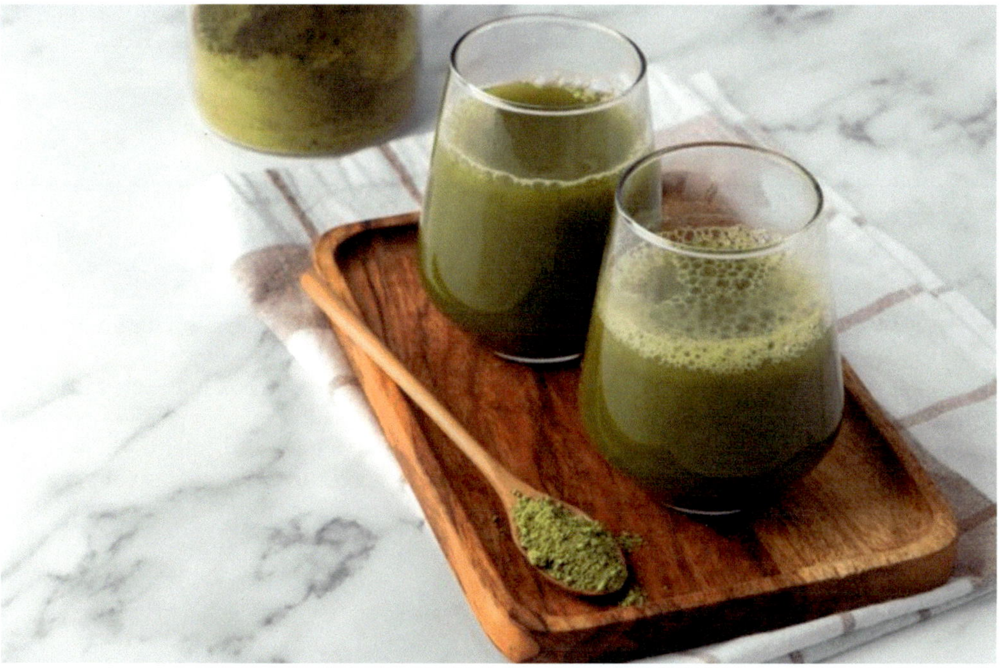

37. Green Tea Matcha Smoothie

Prep.Time: 5 min	**Cook Time:** 0 min	**Serving:** 1	**Beverage pairing:** Green Tea

Ingredients:

- 1 ripe banana
- 1/2 cup unsweetened almond milk
- 1 tablespoon matcha green tea powder
- 1/4 cup plain Greek yogurt
- 1 tablespoon honey or maple syrup (optional)
- Ice cubes (optional)

Preparation:

1. Place all the ingredients in a blender.
2. Blend until smooth and creamy.
3. Add ice cubes if desired and blend again until well combined.
4. Pour into a glass and serve immediately.

Nutrient Facts (per serving):

- Calories: 150
- Carbohydrates: 25g
- Fat: 3g
- Protein: 6g

38. Spinach and Mushroom Breakfast Burrito

Prep.Time:	Cook Time:	Serving:	Beverage pairing:
10 min	10 min	1	Herbal Tea

Ingredients:

- 1 large whole wheat tortilla
- 2 large eggs, scrambled
- 1/4 cup sliced mushrooms
- 1/4 cup baby spinach leaves
- 2 tablespoons shredded cheddar cheese (reduced-fat)
- Salt and pepper to taste
- Cooking spray

Preparation:

1. Heat a skillet over medium heat and lightly coat with cooking spray.
2. Sauté sliced mushrooms until they release their moisture and become tender, about 3-4 minutes.
3. Add baby spinach leaves to the skillet and cook until wilted, about 1-2 minutes.
4. Add scrambled eggs to the skillet and cook until set, stirring occasionally.
5. Season with salt and pepper to taste.
6. Place the scrambled egg mixture onto the center of the whole wheat tortilla.
7. Sprinkle shredded cheddar cheese over the egg mixture.
8. Fold the sides of the tortilla over the filling to create a burrito.

Nutrient Facts (per serving):

- Calories: 300
- Carbohydrates: 25g
- Fat: 15g
- Protein: 18g

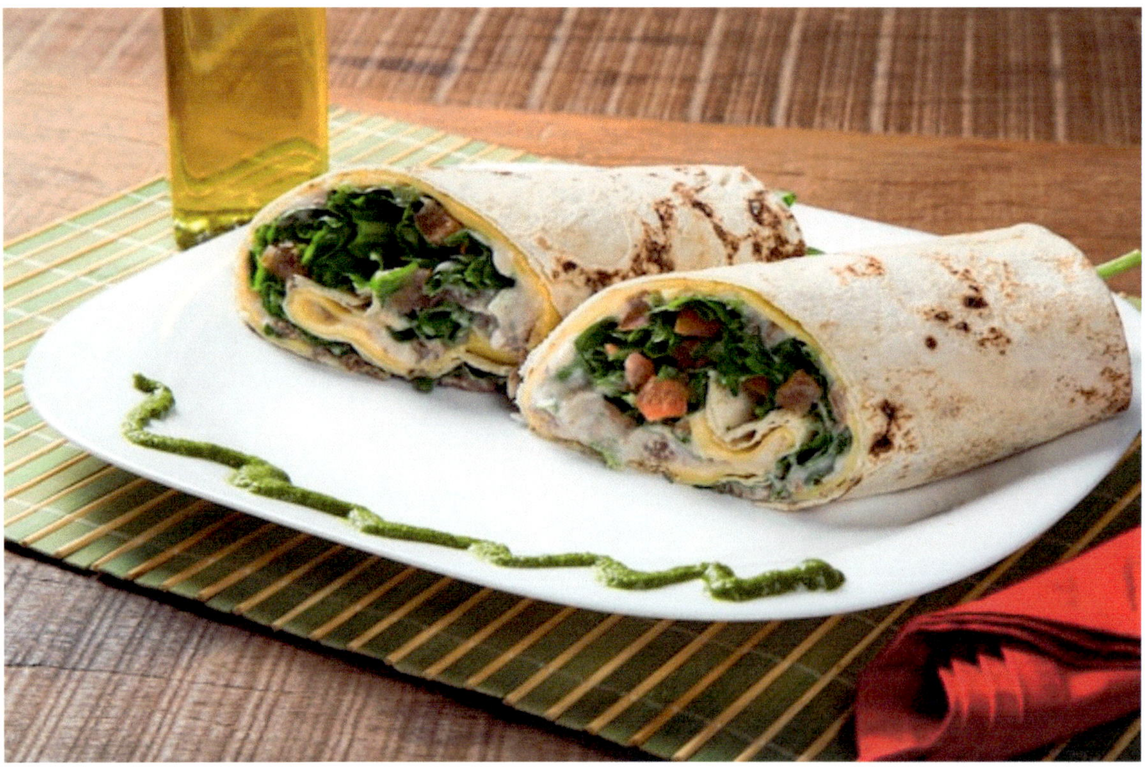

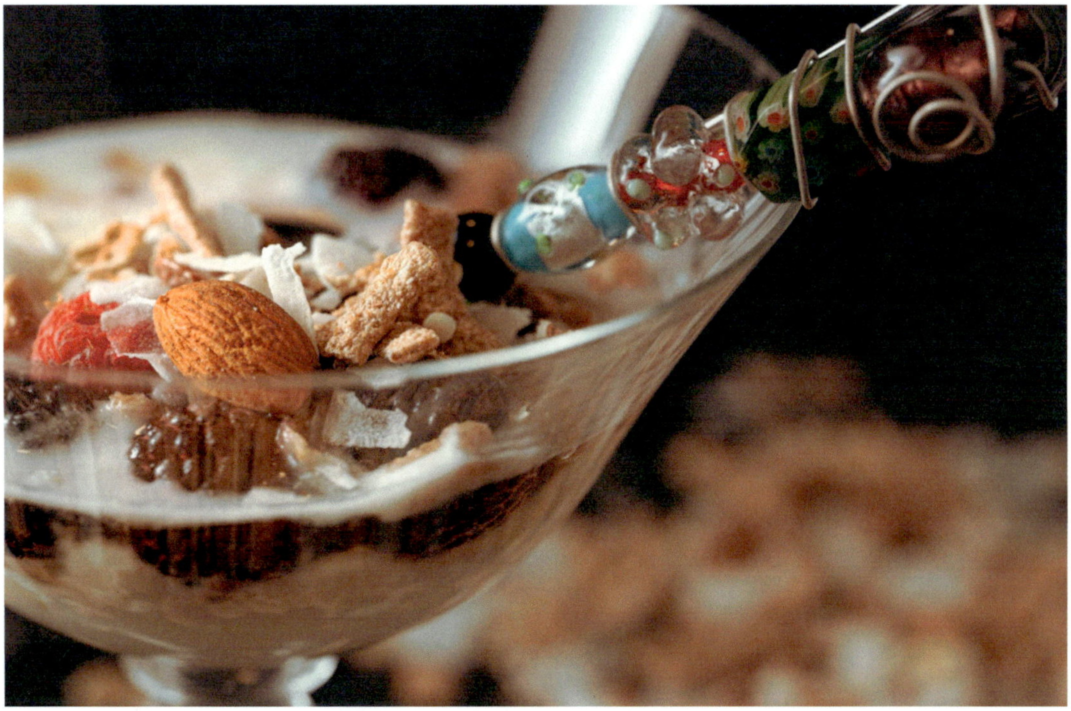

39. Coconut Almond Granola with Yogurt

Prep.Time: 10 min

Cook Time: 20-25 min

Serving: 2

Beverage pairing: Herbal Tea

Ingredients:

- 1/2 cup rolled oats
- 1/4 cup shredded coconut (unsweetened)
- 1/4 cup chopped almonds
- 1 tablespoon honey or maple syrup
- 1/2 teaspoon vanilla extract
- 1/4 teaspoon cinnamon
- 1/4 cup Greek yogurt (unsweetened)
- 1/4 cup mixed berries (such as strawberries, blueberries, raspberries)

Preparation:

1. Preheat the oven to 300°F (150°C) and line a baking sheet with parchment paper.
2. In a bowl, mix together rolled oats, shredded coconut, chopped almonds, honey or maple syrup, vanilla extract, and cinnamon until well combined.
3. Spread the mixture evenly onto the prepared baking sheet.
4. Bake for 20-25 minutes or until golden brown, stirring halfway through.
5. Allow the granola to cool completely before serving.
6. Serve with Greek yogurt and mixed berries.

Nutrient Facts (per serving):

- Calories: 250
- Carbohydrates: 25g
- Fat: 15g
- Protein: 8g

40. Orange Cranberry Overnight Oats

Prep.Time: 5 min	Cook Time: 0 min	Serving: 1	Beverage pairing: Herbal Tea

Ingredients:

- 1/2 cup rolled oats
- 1/2 cup unsweetened almond milk
- 1/4 cup fresh orange juice
- Zest of 1 orange
- 2 tablespoons dried cranberries
- 1 tablespoon honey or maple syrup (optional)

Preparation:

1. In a jar or container, combine rolled oats, almond milk, orange juice, orange zest, dried cranberries, and honey or maple syrup (if using). Stir well.
2. Cover the jar/container and refrigerate overnight or for at least 4 hours.
3. In the morning, give the oats a stir and enjoy cold.

Nutrient Facts (per serving):

- Calories: 250
- Carbohydrates: 40g
- Fat: 6g
- Protein: 6g

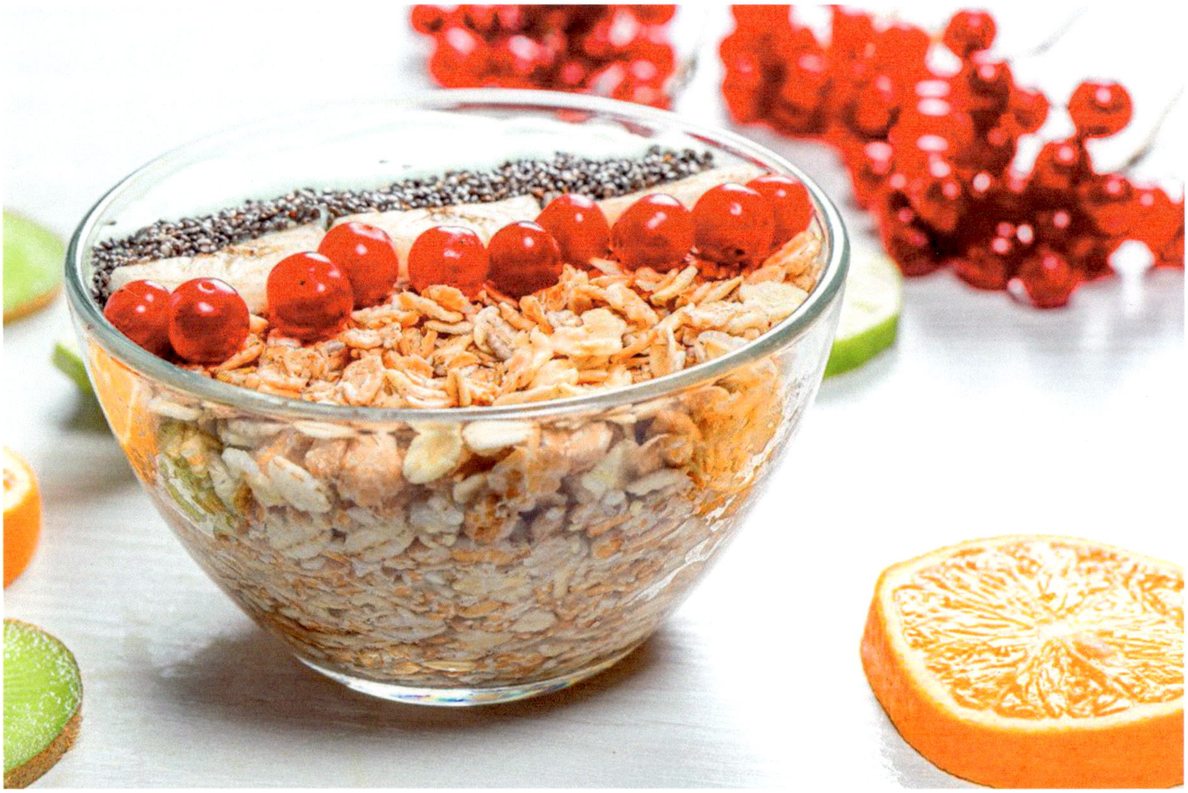

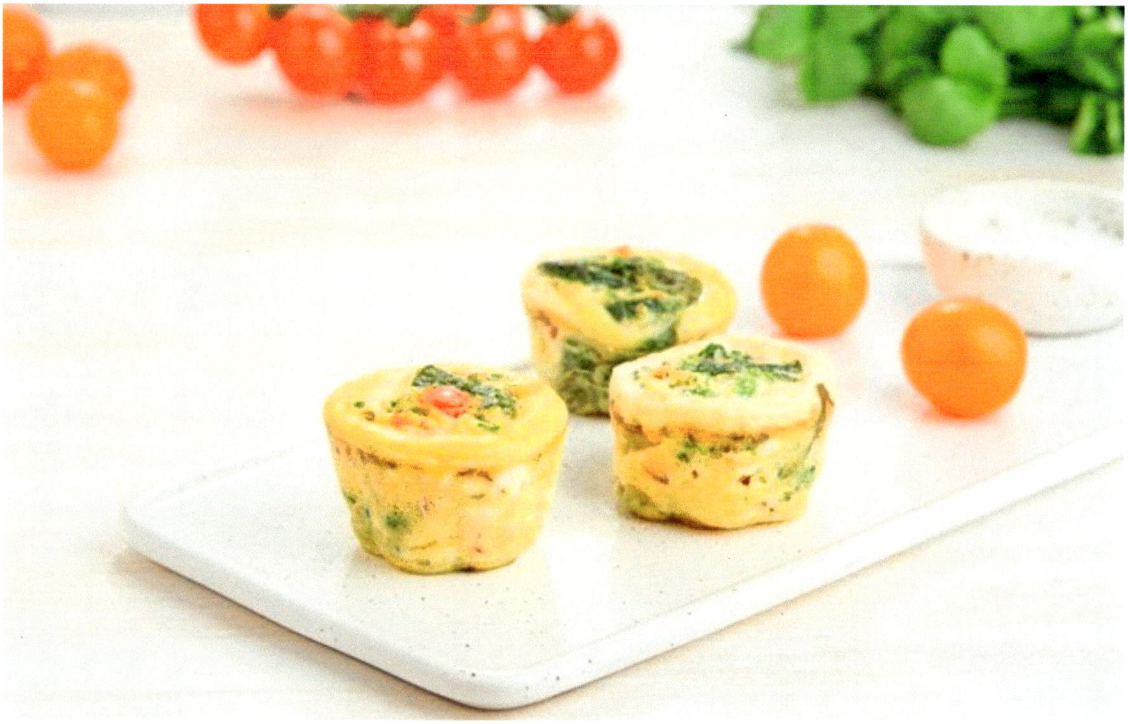

41. Broccoli and Cheddar Egg Cups

Prep.Time:	Cook Time:	Serving:	Beverage pairing:
10 min	15-18 min	2	Herbal Tea

Ingredients:

- 4 large eggs
- 1/2 cup chopped broccoli florets
- 1/4 cup shredded cheddar cheese (reduced-fat)
- Salt and pepper to taste
- Cooking spray

Preparation:

1. Preheat the oven to 350°F (175°C) and grease a muffin tin with cooking spray.
2. In a bowl, beat the eggs and season with salt and pepper.
3. Divide chopped broccoli florets evenly among the muffin cups.
4. Pour the beaten eggs over the broccoli in each muffin cup, filling about 3/4 full.
5. Sprinkle shredded cheddar cheese on top of each egg cup.
6. Bake for 15-18 minutes or until the eggs are set and the tops are golden brown.
7. Allow the egg cups to cool for a few minutes before removing them from the muffin tin.

Nutritional Facts (per serving - 2 egg cups):

- Calories: 200
- Carbohydrates: 4g
- Fat: 14g
- Protein: 15g

42. Chocolate Protein Pancakes

Prep.Time:	Cook Time:	Serving:	Beverage pairing:
10 min	10 min	1	Almond Milk

Ingredients:

- 1/2 cup oats
- 1/2 banana, mashed
- 1 scoop chocolate protein powder
- 1/4 cup unsweetened almond milk
- 1 egg
- 1 tablespoon cocoa powder
- 1/2 teaspoon baking powder
- Cooking spray

Preparation:

1. In a blender, combine oats, mashed banana, chocolate protein powder, almond milk, egg, cocoa powder, and baking powder. Blend until smooth.
2. Heat a non-stick skillet over medium heat and lightly coat with cooking spray.
3. Pour the pancake batter onto the skillet to form pancakes of desired size.
4. Cook for 2-3 minutes on each side until golden brown and cooked through.
5. Serve hot with your choice of toppings, such as fresh berries or a drizzle of honey.

Nutrient Facts (per serving):

- Calories: 300
- Carbohydrates: 30g
- Fat: 8g
- Protein: 25g

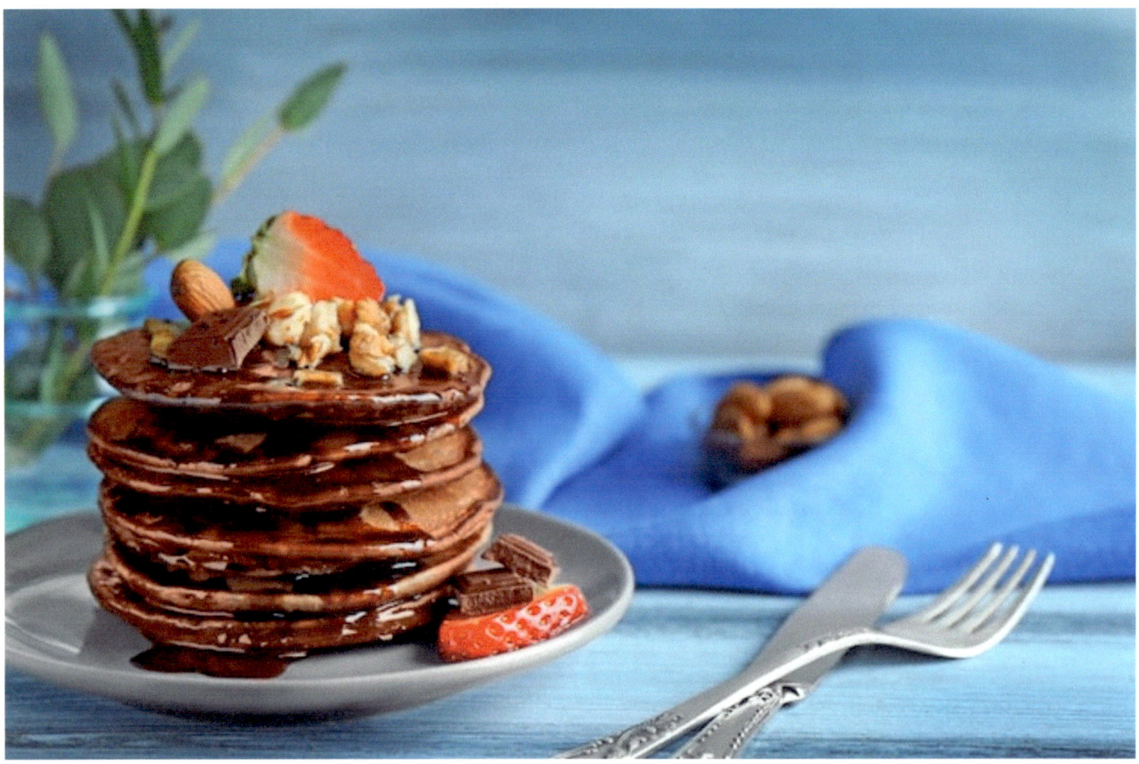

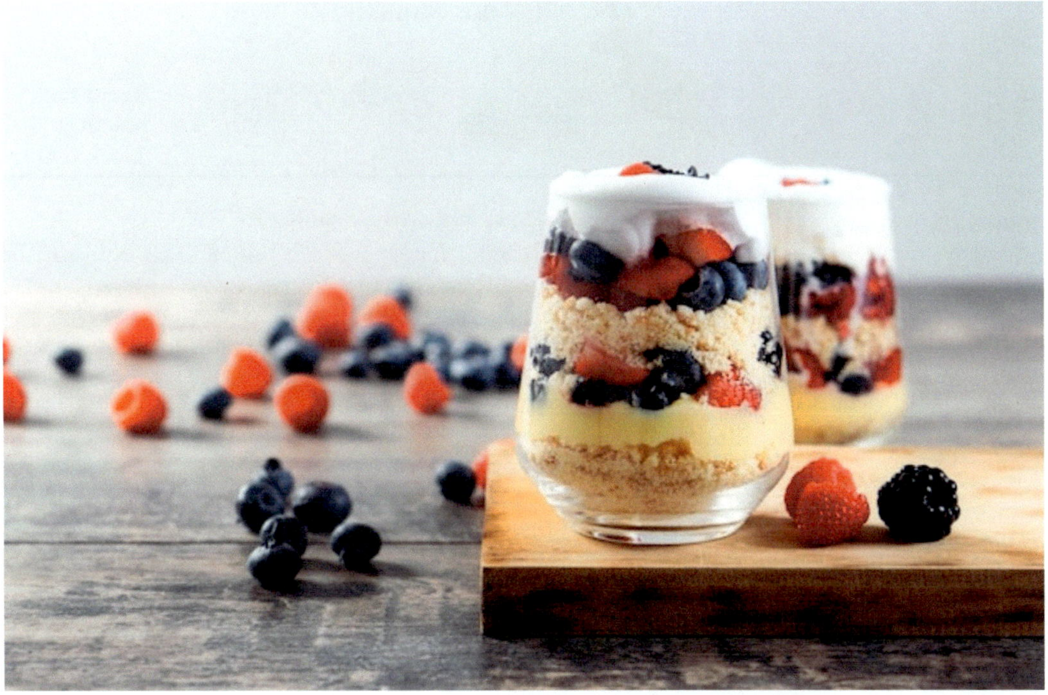

43. Mixed Berry Quinoa Parfait

Prep.Time:	Cook Time:	Serving:	Beverage pairing:
5 min	0 min	1	Green Tea

Ingredients:

- 1/2 cup cooked quinoa
- 1/2 cup mixed berries (such as strawberries, blueberries, raspberries)
- 1/4 cup Greek yogurt (unsweetened)
- 1 tablespoon chopped nuts (such as almonds or walnuts)
- 1 teaspoon honey or maple syrup (optional)

Preparation:

1. In a glass or bowl, layer cooked quinoa, mixed berries, Greek yogurt, and chopped nuts.
2. Drizzle with honey or maple syrup if desired.
3. Repeat the layers until all ingredients are used.
4. Serve chilled.

Nutritional Facts (per serving):

- Calories: 250
- Carbohydrates: 35g
- Fat: 6g
- Protein: 10g

44. Mexican Shakshuka

Prep.Time: 15 min	**Cook Time:** 20 min	**Serving:** 2	**Beverage pairing:** Black Coffee

Ingredients:

- 1 tablespoon olive oil
- 1/2 onion, diced
- 1 bell pepper, diced
- 2 cloves garlic, minced
- 1 teaspoon ground cumin
- 1 teaspoon smoked paprika
- 1/2 teaspoon chili powder
- 1 can (14 oz) diced tomatoes
- 4 eggs
- Salt and pepper to taste
- Fresh cilantro for garnish (optional)
- Crumbled feta cheese for garnish (optional)
- Sliced avocado for serving (optional)

Preparation:

1. Heat olive oil in a skillet over medium heat.
2. Add diced onion and bell pepper to the skillet. Cook until softened, about 5 minutes.
3. Add minced garlic, ground cumin, smoked paprika, and chili powder to the skillet. Cook for an additional 1-2 minutes until fragrant.
4. Pour diced tomatoes into the skillet and simmer for 5-7 minutes until the sauce thickens slightly.
5. Using a spoon, create small wells in the tomato mixture and crack eggs into the wells.
6. Cover the skillet and cook for 5-7 minutes until the egg whites are set but the yolks are still runny.
7. Season with salt and pepper to taste.
8. Garnish with fresh cilantro and crumbled feta cheese if desired.
9. Serve hot with sliced avocado on the side and whole grain bread for dipping.

Nutrient Facts (per serving):

- Calories: 250
- Carbohydrates: 15g
- Fat: 15g
- Protein: 12g

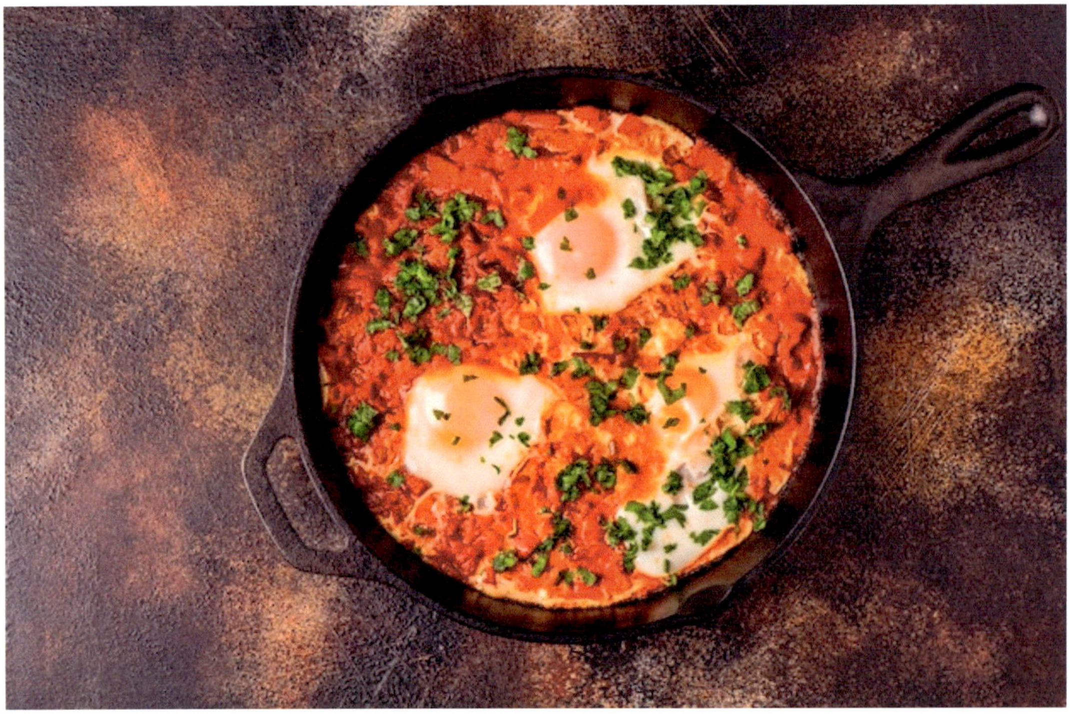

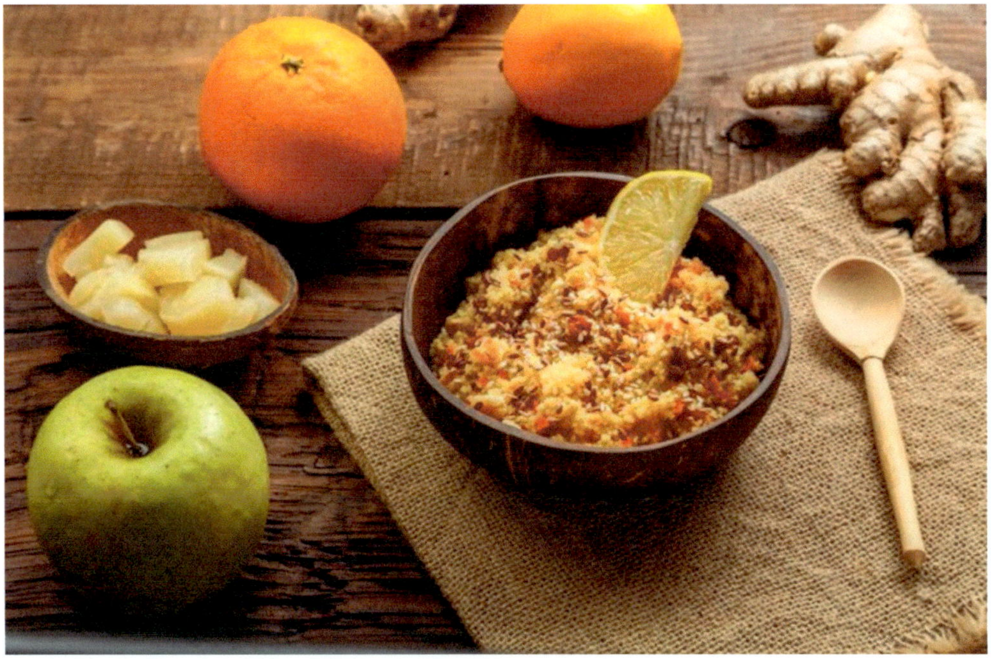

45. Apple Pecan Breakfast Couscous

Prep.Time: 10 min	**Cook Time:** 5 min	**Serving:** 1	**Beverage pairing:** Herbal Tea

Ingredients:

- 1/2 cup whole wheat couscous
- 1/2 cup unsweetened almond milk
- 1/2 apple, diced
- 2 tablespoons chopped pecans
- 1 tablespoon honey or maple syrup
- 1/4 teaspoon cinnamon
- Pinch of salt

Preparation:

1. In a small saucepan, bring almond milk to a boil.
2. Stir in whole wheat couscous, diced apple, chopped pecans, honey or maple syrup, cinnamon, and a pinch of salt.
3. Cover the saucepan and remove it from heat. Let it sit for 5 minutes.
4. Fluff the couscous with a fork and serve hot.

Nutritional Facts (per serving):

- Calories: 300
- Carbohydrates: 45g
- Fat: 8g
- Protein: 6g

46. Avocado and Black Bean Breakfast Bowl

Prep.Time:	Cook Time:	Serving:	Beverage pairing:
10 min	10 min	1	Black Coffee

Ingredients:

- 1/2 avocado, sliced
- 1/4 cup black beans, cooked
- 2 large eggs, cooked to your preference (scrambled, fried, or poached)
- 1/4 cup diced tomatoes
- 1/4 cup diced red onions
- Fresh cilantro for garnish (optional)
- Lime wedges for serving (optional)
- Salt and pepper to taste

Preparation:

1. Arrange sliced avocado, cooked black beans, and cooked eggs in a bowl.
2. Top with diced tomatoes and diced red onions.
3. Garnish with fresh cilantro if desired.
4. Season with salt and pepper to taste.
5. Serve with lime wedges on the side for added flavor.

Nutrient Facts (per serving):

- Calories: 300
- Carbohydrates: 20g
- Fat: 18g
- Protein: 15g

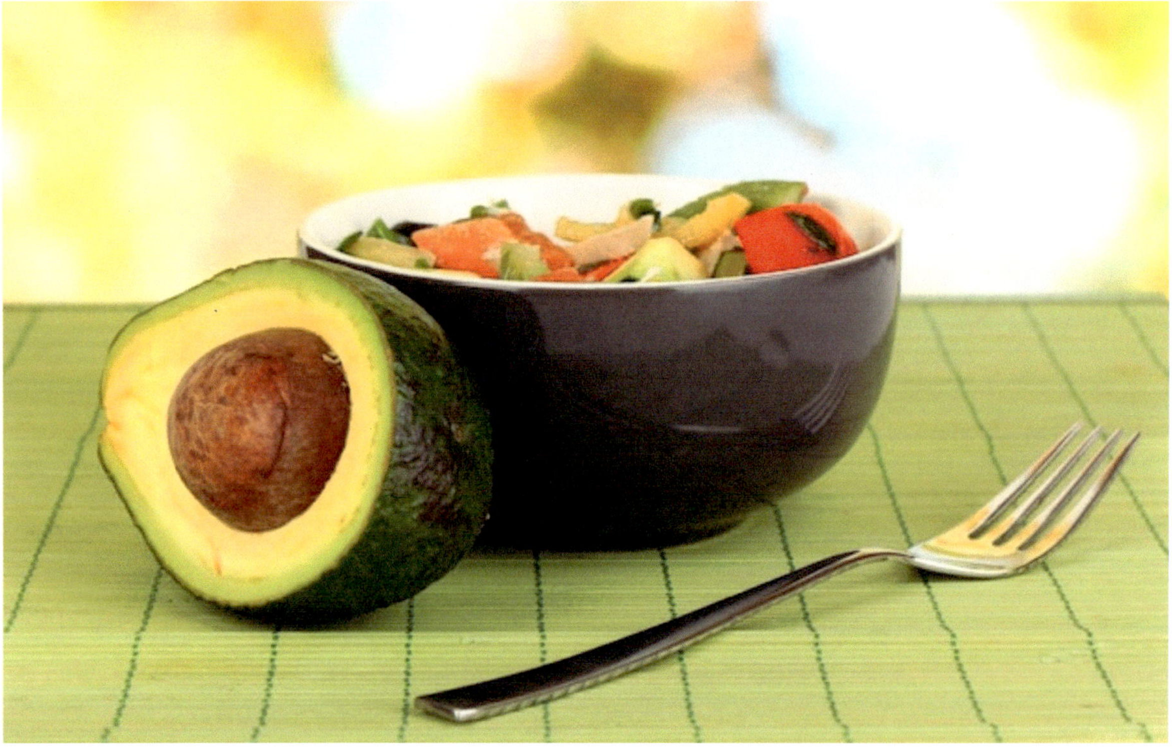

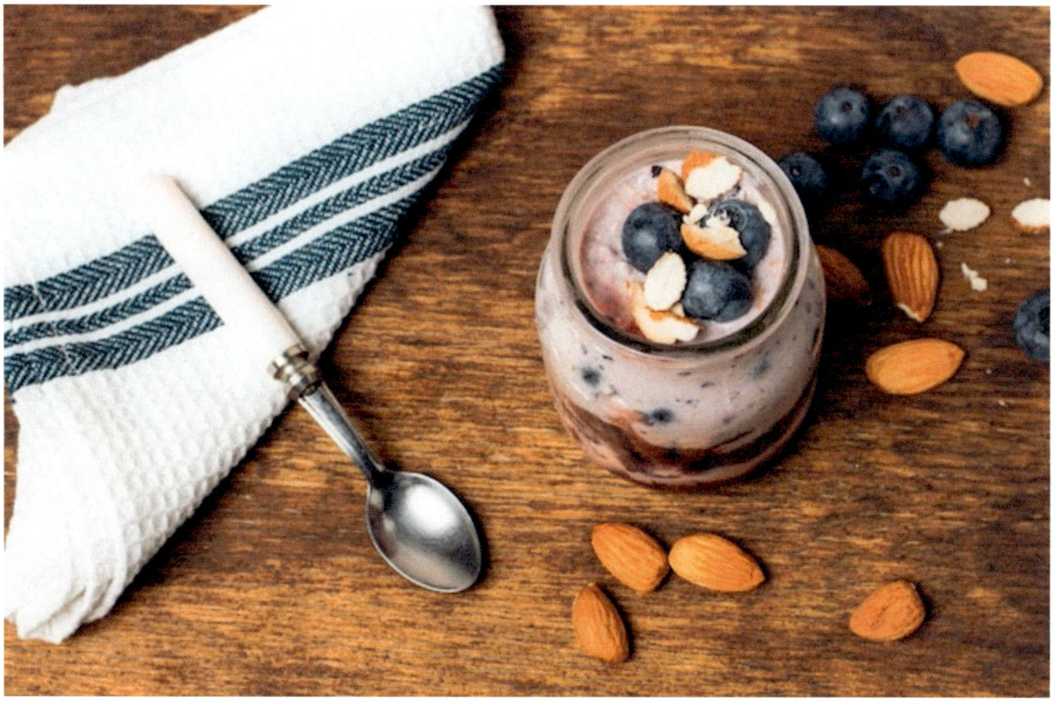

47. Vanilla Almond Chia Pudding

Prep.Time: 5 min | **Cook Time:** 0 min | **Serving:** 1 | **Beverage pairing:** Herbal Tea

Ingredients:

- 2 tablespoons chia seeds
- 1/2 cup unsweetened almond milk
- 1/4 teaspoon vanilla extract
- 1 tablespoon sliced almonds
- 1 teaspoon honey or maple syrup (optional)

Preparation:

1. In a bowl, mix together chia seeds, almond milk, and vanilla extract.
2. Cover and refrigerate for at least 2 hours or overnight, allowing the chia seeds to gel and thicken.
3. Before serving, top with sliced almonds and drizzle with honey or maple syrup if desired.

Nutritional Facts (per serving):

- Calories: 150
- Carbohydrates: 10g
- Fat: 9g
- Protein: 5g

48. Almond Joy Smoothie Bowl

Prep.Time: 5 min

Cook Time: 0 min

Serving: 1

Beverage pairing: Herbal Tea

Ingredients:

- 1 ripe banana, frozen
- 1/2 cup unsweetened almond milk
- 1 tablespoon cocoa powder
- 1 tablespoon almond butter
- 1 tablespoon shredded coconut (unsweetened)
- 1 tablespoon sliced almonds
- 1 teaspoon honey or maple syrup (optional)

Preparation:

1. In a blender, combine frozen banana, almond milk, cocoa powder, and almond butter.
2. Blend until smooth and creamy.
3. Pour the smoothie into a bowl.
4. Top with shredded coconut, sliced almonds, and drizzle with honey or maple syrup if desired.

Nutrient Facts (per serving):

- Calories: 300
- Carbohydrates: 30g
- Fat: 15g
- Protein: 6g

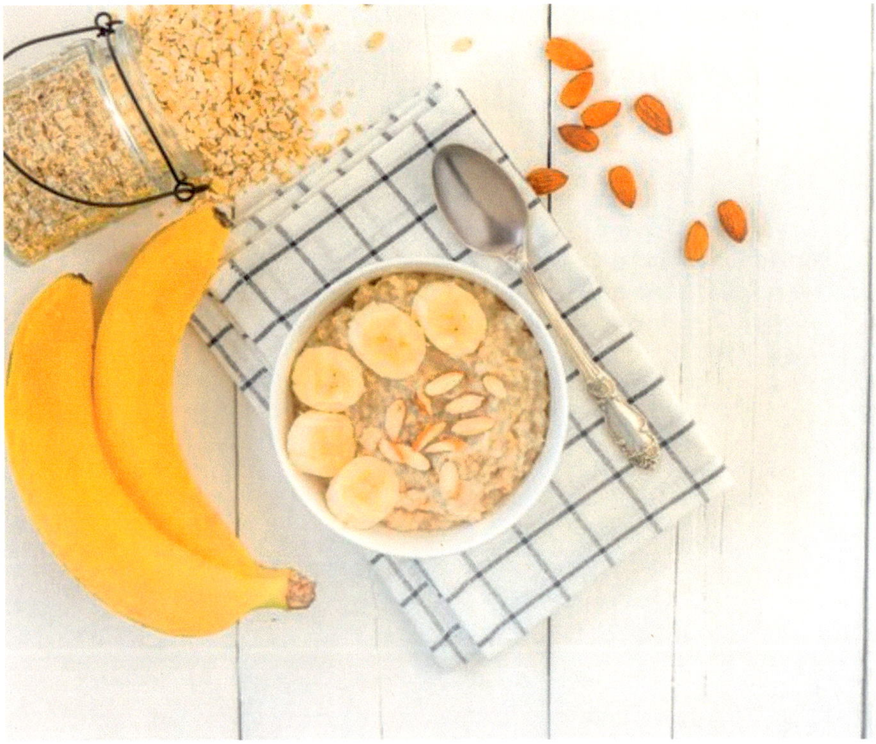

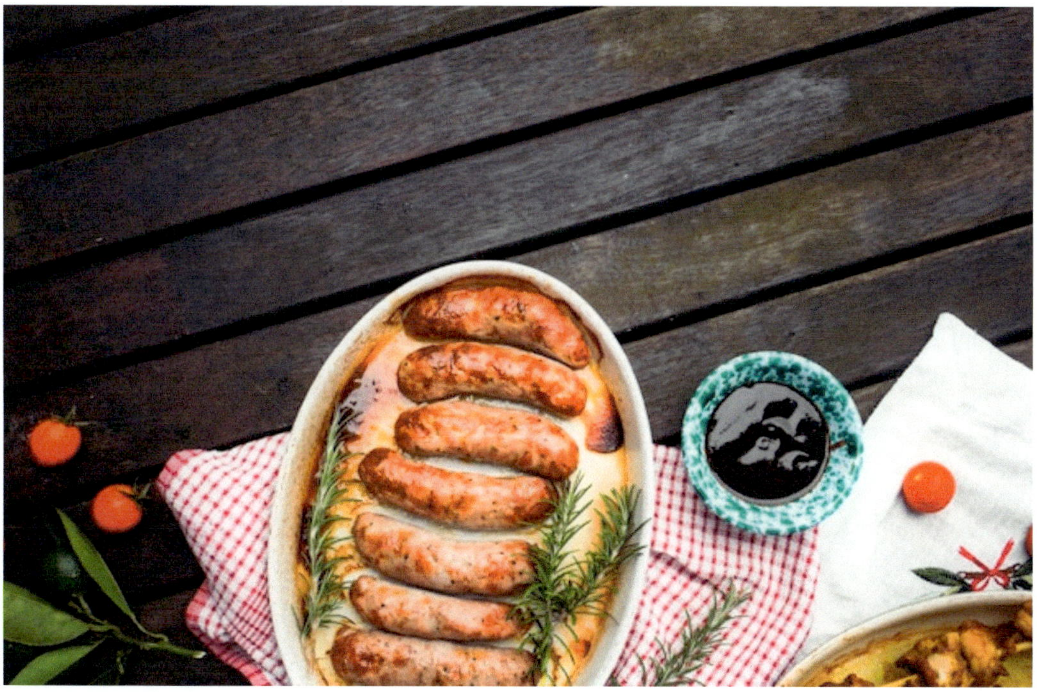

49. Turkey Sausage Breakfast Casserole

Prep.Time: 15 min

Cook Time: 25-30 min

Serving: 6

Beverage pairing: Herbal Tea

Ingredients:

- 6 slices whole wheat bread, cubed
- 6 ounces turkey sausage, cooked and crumbled
- 1 cup diced bell peppers (any color)
- 1 cup diced onions
- 1 cup baby spinach leaves
- 1 cup shredded cheddar cheese (reduced-fat)
- 6 large eggs
- 1 cup unsweetened almond milk
- 1 teaspoon dried thyme
- Salt and pepper to taste
- Cooking spray

Preparation:

1. Preheat the oven to 350°F (175°C) and lightly grease a 9x13-inch baking dish with cooking spray.
2. In a large bowl, combine cubed whole wheat bread, cooked turkey sausage, diced bell peppers, diced onions, baby spinach leaves, and shredded cheddar cheese. Mix well.
3. Transfer the mixture to the prepared baking dish, spreading it out evenly.
4. In another bowl, whisk together eggs, almond milk, dried thyme, salt, and pepper.
5. Pour the egg mixture over the bread mixture in the baking dish, ensuring it is evenly distributed.
6. Bake for 25-30 minutes or until the eggs are set and the top is golden brown.
7. Allow the casserole to cool for a few minutes before slicing and serving.

Nutritional Facts (per serving):

- Calories: 300
- Carbohydrates: 15g
- Fat: 15g
- Protein: 25g

50. Peach Cobbler Overnight Oats

Prep.Time: 5 min | **Cook Time:** 0 min | **Serving:** 1 | **Beverage pairing:** Black Coffee

Ingredients:

- 1/2 cup rolled oats
- 1/2 cup unsweetened almond milk
- 1/2 peach, diced
- 1 tablespoon chopped pecans
- 1 tablespoon maple syrup
- 1/4 teaspoon cinnamon

Preparation:

1. In a jar or container, combine rolled oats, almond milk, diced peach, chopped pecans, maple syrup, and cinnamon. Stir well.
2. Cover the jar/container and refrigerate overnight or for at least 4 hours.
3. In the morning, give the oats a stir and enjoy cold.

Nutrient Facts (per serving):

- Calories: 250
- Carbohydrates: 35g
- Fat: 8g
- Protein: 6g

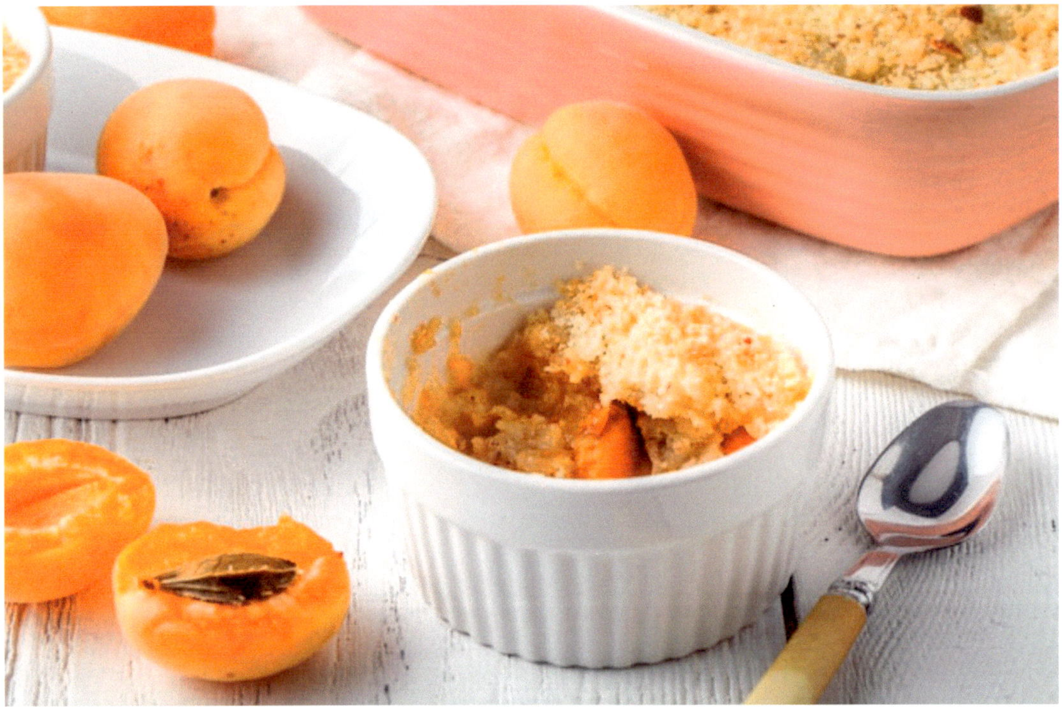

Your Kindness is Key

Share Your Experience, Share Your Strength

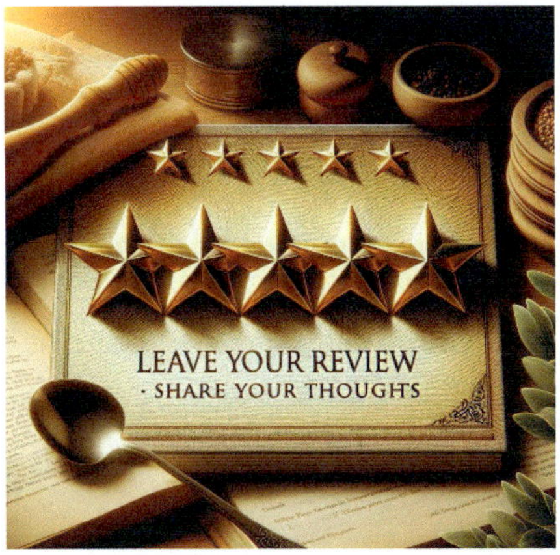

"Helping one person might not change the whole world, but it could change the world for one person." - Anonymous

---

Do you remember what it was like when you first heard the words "Type 2 Diabetes?" Perhaps it felt like a mountain you weren't sure you could climb.

Maybe it was daunting, thinking about the changes you'd have to make in your life, especially with your diet. It's a journey many embark on feeling uncertain and alone.

But you've found a companion on this journey, haven't you? Type 2 Diabetes Cookbook Beginner's Quick & Easy Recipes for Delicious Diabetes Diets by Lily Anders has been with you, offering guidance, delicious recipes, and a sense of control over your diabetes that perhaps you didn't feel before.

Imagine if you could light the path for someone just starting on this journey. Someone who feels lost in the sea of information, unsure of where to turn for reliable, practical advice on managing their diabetes through diet. Your experience, shared through a review, could be the beacon they need.

This isn't just about leaving a review; it's about extending a hand, offering support, and sharing the strength that comes from knowledge and community. Your words could help another person find their footing, making their journey a bit easier and less lonely.

So, here's my humble request on behalf of a fellow journeyer you've yet to meet:

Please take a moment to share your experience with the book. Your insights could be the very thing another person needs to hear to take that first, brave step toward a healthier, happier life with diabetes. Your review, a simple act of kindness, asks for nothing in return yet offers immeasurable value.

To leave your review, just follow this link:

https://www.amazon.com/review/create-review/?ie=UTF8&channel=glance-detail&asin=1963939298

If the thought of helping another soul on their diabetes journey warms your heart, then you're exactly who I hoped to reach with this book. Welcome to a community where kindness, support, and shared victories pave the way to a better life.

I'm beyond grateful for your help in spreading the word and even more excited to continue providing you with the knowledge and recipes to make managing diabetes not just manageable, but enjoyable.

Click the QR Code Here!

Thank you from the deepest places in my heart. Your generosity makes all the difference.

Lily Anders

P.S. - Sharing is caring, they say. If you believe this book has brought value to your life and could do the same for someone else, consider sharing it with them. It's another beautiful way to change a life, one meal at a time.

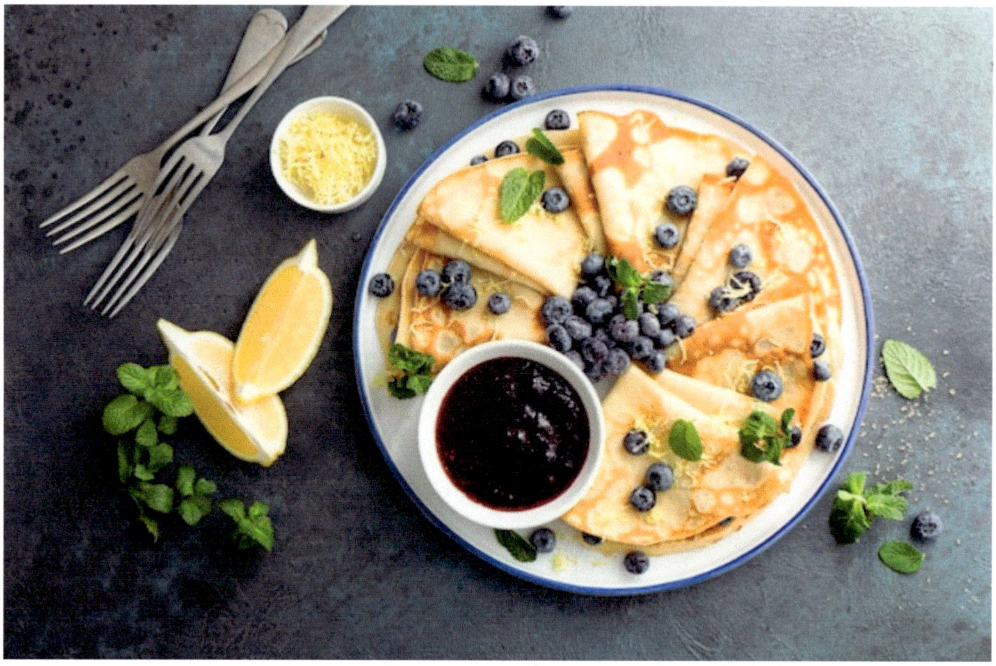

51. Blueberry Lemon Ricotta Pancakes

Prep.Time: 10 min	Cook Time: 10 min	Serving: 2	Beverage pairing: Herbal Tea

Ingredients:

- 1/2 cup whole wheat flour
- 1/2 teaspoon baking powder
- 1/4 teaspoon baking soda
- Pinch of salt
- 1/2 cup part-skim ricotta cheese
- 1/4 cup unsweetened almond milk
- 1 large egg
- 1 tablespoon honey or maple syrup
- Zest of 1 lemon
- 1/2 cup fresh blueberries
- Cooking spray

Preparation:

1. In a large bowl, whisk together whole wheat flour, baking powder, baking soda, and salt.
2. In another bowl, mix ricotta cheese, almond milk, egg, honey or maple syrup, and lemon zest until well combined.
3. Pour the wet ingredients into the dry ingredients and stir until just combined.
4. Gently fold in fresh blueberries.
5. Heat a non-stick skillet or griddle over medium heat and lightly coat with cooking spray.
6. Pour 1/4 cup of batter onto the skillet for each pancake.
7. Cook for 2-3 minutes on each side until golden brown and cooked through.
8. Serve hot with your choice of toppings, such as extra blueberries or a drizzle of honey.

Nutritional Facts (per serving - 2 pancakes):

- Calories: 300
- Carbohydrates: 35g
- Fat: 10g
- Protein: 15g

52. Veggie and Feta Breakfast Wrap

Prep.Time:	Cook Time:	Serving:	Beverage pairing:
10 min	10 min	1	Black Coffee

Ingredients:

- 1 whole wheat tortilla
- 2 large eggs, scrambled
- 1/4 cup diced tomatoes
- 1/4 cup diced bell peppers (any color)
- 1/4 cup baby spinach leaves
- 2 tablespoons crumbled feta cheese
- Salt and pepper to taste
- Cooking spray

Preparation:

1. Heat a skillet over medium heat and lightly coat with cooking spray.
2. Add diced tomatoes and diced bell peppers to the skillet. Cook until softened, about 3-4 minutes.
3. Add baby spinach leaves to the skillet and cook until wilted, about 1-2 minutes.
4. Add scrambled eggs to the skillet and cook until set, stirring occasionally.
5. Season with salt and pepper to taste.
6. Warm the whole wheat tortilla in the microwave for 10-15 seconds.
7. Place the scrambled egg mixture in the center of the tortilla.
8. Sprinkle crumbled feta cheese over the egg mixture.
9. Fold the sides of the tortilla over the filling to create a wrap.

Nutrient Facts (per serving):

- Calories: 300
- Carbohydrates: 25g
- Fat: 15g
- Protein: 18g

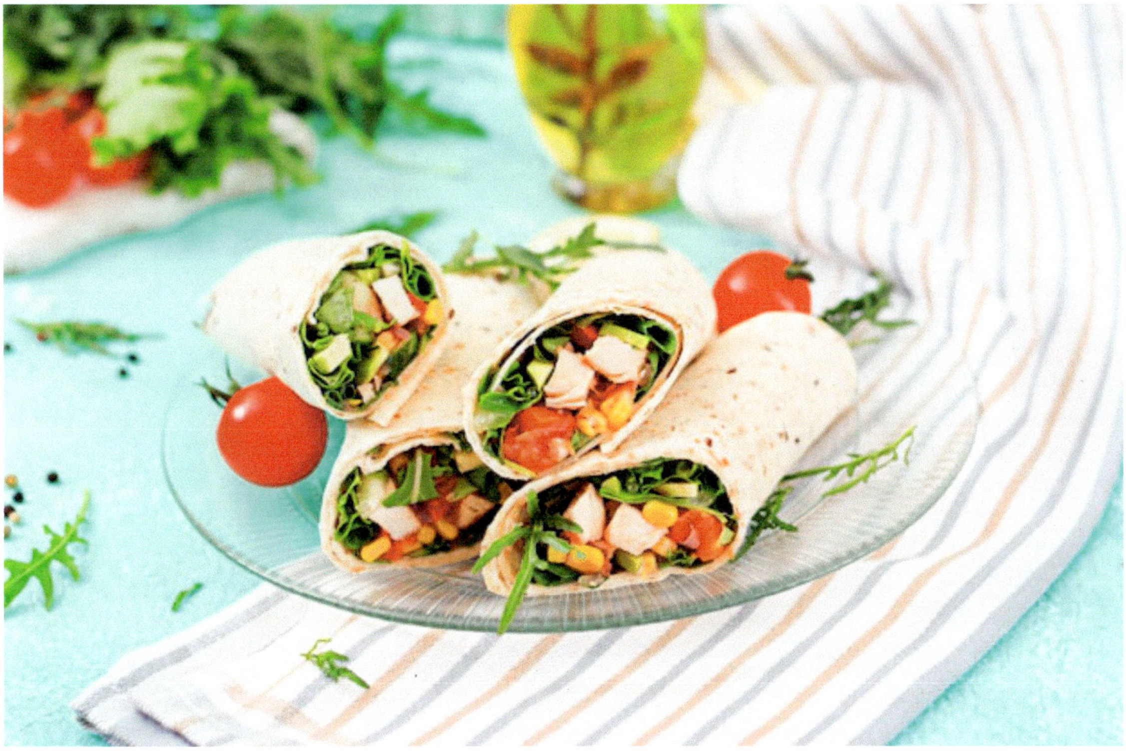

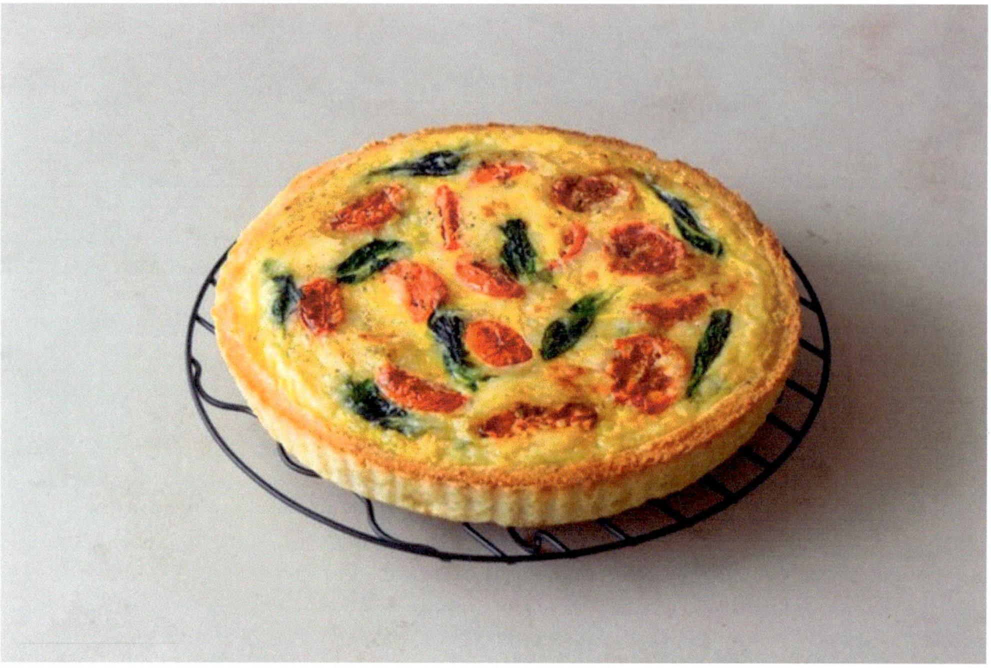

53. Tomato Basil Quiche

Prep.Time:	Cook Time:	Serving:	Beverage pairing:
10 min	35-40 min	6	Herbal Tea

Ingredients:

- 1 pie crust (store-bought or homemade)
- 4 large eggs
- 1 cup milk (any type, such as dairy or almond milk)
- 1 cup diced tomatoes
- 1/2 cup shredded mozzarella cheese
- 1/4 cup chopped fresh basil
- Salt and pepper to taste
- Cooking spray

Preparation:

1. Preheat the oven to 375°F (190°C).
2. Place the pie crust in a pie dish and press it down evenly.
3. In a bowl, whisk together eggs and milk until well combined. Season with salt and pepper.
4. Spread diced tomatoes, shredded mozzarella cheese, and chopped fresh basil evenly over the pie crust.
5. Pour the egg mixture over the fillings in the pie crust.
6. Bake for 35-40 minutes or until the quiche is set and the crust is golden brown.
7. Allow the quiche to cool for a few minutes before slicing and serving.

Nutritional Facts (per serving):

- Calories: 250
- Carbohydrates: 15g
- Fat: 15g
- Protein: 12g

54. Mango Pineapple Smoothie

Prep.Time: 5 min	**Cook Time:** 0 min	**Serving:** 1	**Beverage pairing:** Herbal Tea

Ingredients:

- 1 cup frozen mango chunks
- 1/2 cup frozen pineapple chunks
- 1/2 cup Greek yogurt (unsweetened)
- 1/2 cup unsweetened almond milk
- 1 tablespoon honey or maple syrup (optional)
- Ice cubes (optional)

Preparation:

1. In a blender, combine frozen mango chunks, frozen pineapple chunks, Greek yogurt, almond milk, and honey or maple syrup (if using).
2. Blend until smooth and creamy.
3. Add ice cubes if desired and blend again until well combined.
4. Pour into a glass and serve immediately.

Nutrient Facts (per serving):

- Calories: 200
- Carbohydrates: 30g
- Fat: 3g
- Protein: 15g

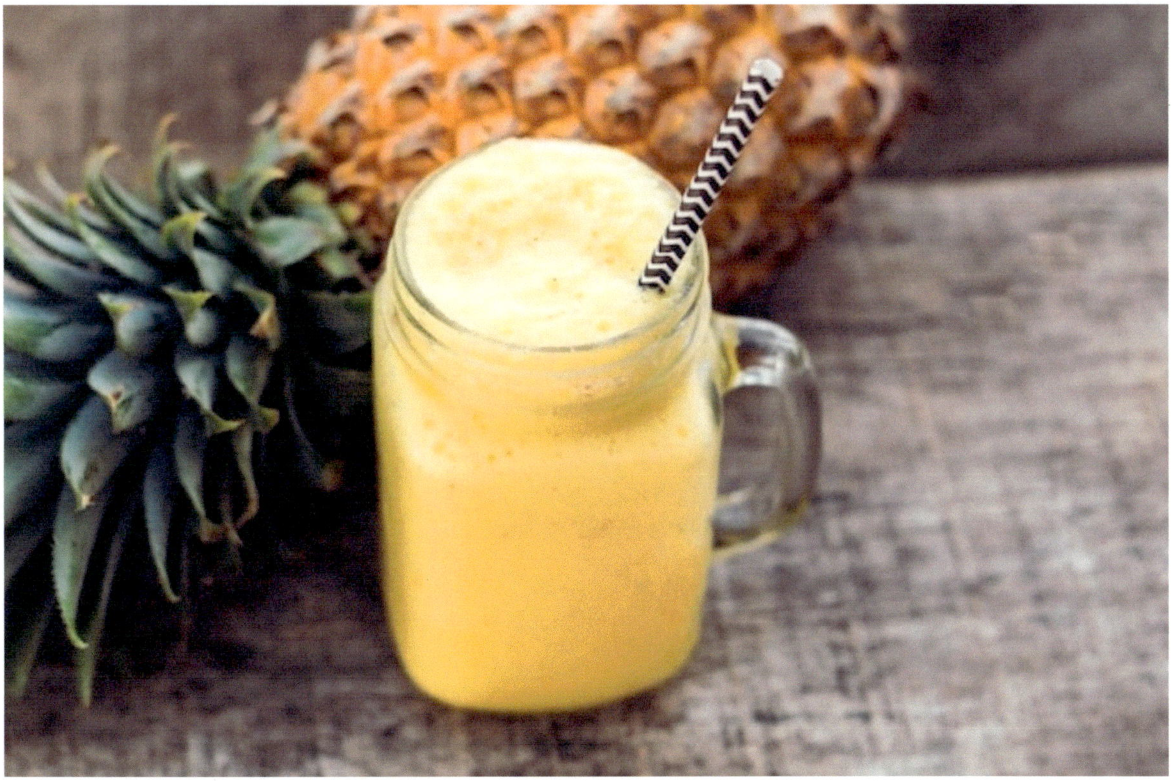

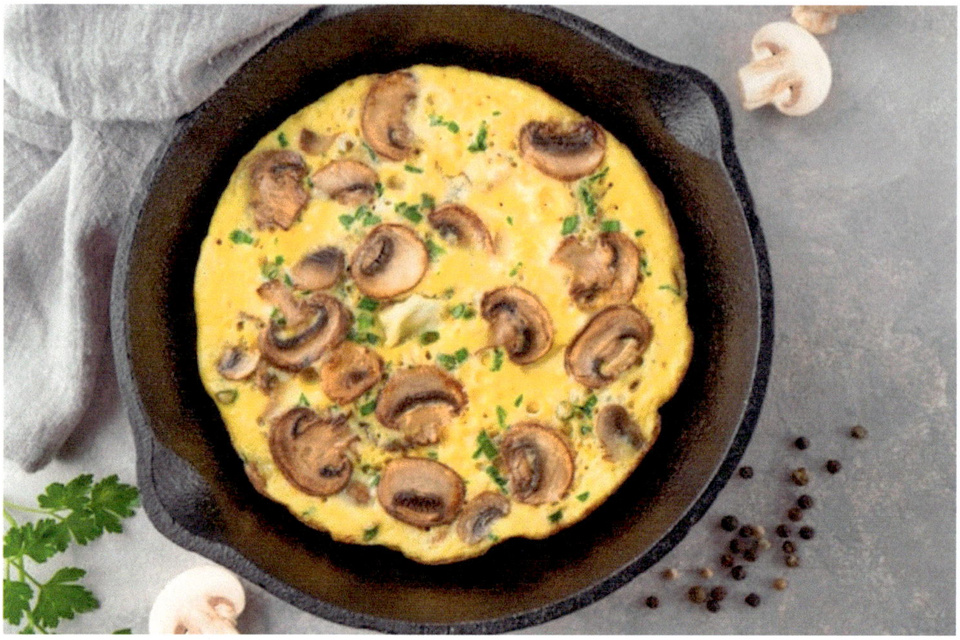

55. Caramelized Onion and Mushroom Omelette

Prep.Time: 10 min	Cook Time: 20 min	Serving: 1	Beverage pairing: Black Coffee

Ingredients:

- 2 large eggs
- 1/2 cup sliced mushrooms
- 1/4 cup thinly sliced onions
- 1 tablespoon olive oil
- 1 tablespoon shredded cheddar cheese (reduced-fat)
- Salt and pepper to taste

Preparation:

1. Heat olive oil in a skillet over medium heat.
2. Add thinly sliced onions to the skillet and cook until caramelized, about 10-15 minutes, stirring occasionally.
3. Add sliced mushrooms to the skillet and cook until softened, about 5 minutes.
4. In a bowl, beat the eggs and season with salt and pepper.
5. Pour the beaten eggs into the skillet, covering the caramelized onions and mushrooms.
6. Cook until the omelette is set, lifting the edges with a spatula and tilting the skillet to let the uncooked egg flow underneath.
7. Sprinkle shredded cheddar cheese over one half of the omelette.
8. Fold the other half of the omelette over the cheese filling.
9. Slide the omelette onto a plate and serve hot.

Nutritional Facts (per serving):

- Calories: 250
- Carbohydrates: 5g
- Fat: 18g
- Protein: 15g

56. Cranberry Orange Scones

Prep.Time: 15 min

Cook Time: 15-18 min

Serving: 8

Beverage pairing: Herbal Tea

Ingredients:

- 2 cups all-purpose flour
- 1/4 cup granulated sugar
- 1 tablespoon baking powder
- 1/2 teaspoon salt
- Zest of 1 orange
- 1/2 cup cold unsalted butter, cubed
- 1/2 cup dried cranberries
- 1/2 cup milk (any type)
- 1 large egg
- 1 teaspoon vanilla extract

Preparation:

1. Preheat the oven to 400°F (200°C) and line a baking sheet with parchment paper.
2. In a large bowl, whisk together all-purpose flour, granulated sugar, baking powder, salt, and orange zest.
3. Cut in cold unsalted butter using a pastry cutter or fork until the mixture resembles coarse crumbs.
4. Stir in dried cranberries.
5. In a separate bowl, whisk together milk, egg, and vanilla extract.
6. Gradually add the wet ingredients to the dry ingredients, stirring until just combined.
7. Turn the dough out onto a lightly floured surface and knead gently until it comes together.
8. Pat the dough into a circle about 1-inch thick. Cut into 8 wedges.
9. Place the scones onto the prepared baking sheet, leaving space between each one.
10. Bake for 15-18 minutes or until golden brown.
11. Allow the scones to cool on the baking sheet for a few minutes before transferring them to a wire rack to cool completely.

Nutrient Facts (per serving):

- Calories: 250
- Carbohydrates: 30g
- Fat: 12g
- Protein: 4g

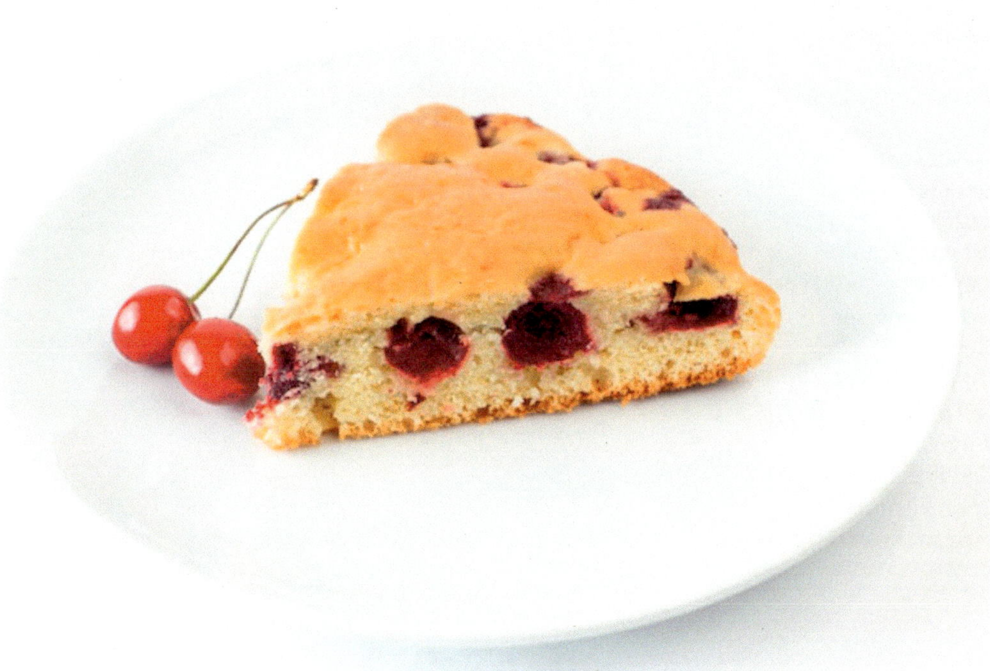

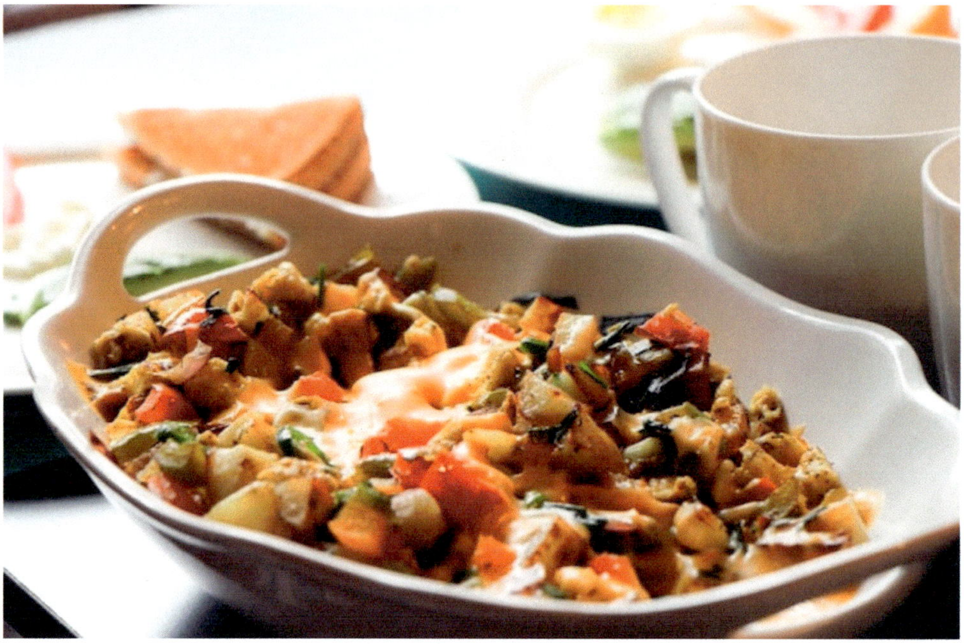

57. Southwest Tofu Scramble

Prep.Time:	Cook Time:	Serving:	Beverage pairing:
10 min	15 min	2	Black Coffee

Ingredients:

- 1/2 block extra-firm tofu, crumbled
- 1/4 cup diced bell peppers (any color)
- 1/4 cup diced onions
- 1/4 cup black beans, drained and rinsed
- 1/4 cup corn kernels (fresh or frozen)
- 1/4 cup diced tomatoes
- 1/4 teaspoon chili powder
- 1/4 teaspoon cumin
- Salt and pepper to taste
- Cooking spray
- Fresh cilantro for garnish (optional)

Preparation:

1. Heat a skillet over medium heat and lightly coat with cooking spray.
2. Add diced bell peppers and diced onions to the skillet. Cook until softened, about 5 minutes.
3. Add crumbled tofu to the skillet and cook for 3-4 minutes, stirring occasionally.
4. Stir in black beans, corn kernels, diced tomatoes, chili powder, cumin, salt, and pepper. Cook for an additional 2-3 minutes until heated through.
5. Garnish with fresh cilantro if desired.
6. Serve hot with sliced avocado on the side.

Nutritional Facts (per serving):

- Calories: 200
- Carbohydrates: 15g
- Fat: 10g
- Protein: 15g

58. Raspberry Coconut Chia Pudding

Prep.Time:	Cook Time:	Serving:	Beverage pairing:
5 min	0 min	1	Black Cofee

Ingredients:

- 2 tablespoons chia seeds
- 1/2 cup coconut milk
- 1/4 cup Greek yogurt (unsweetened)
- 1/4 cup raspberries (fresh or frozen)
- 1 tablespoon shredded coconut (unsweetened)
- 1 teaspoon honey or maple syrup (optional)

Preparation:

1. In a bowl, mix together chia seeds, coconut milk, and Greek yogurt until well combined.
2. Gently fold in raspberries.
3. Cover the bowl and refrigerate for at least 2 hours or overnight, allowing the chia seeds to gel and thicken.
4. Before serving, sprinkle shredded coconut on top and drizzle with honey or maple syrup if desired.

Nutrient Facts (per serving):

- Calories: 200
- Carbohydrates: 15g
- Fat: 12g
- Protein: 6g

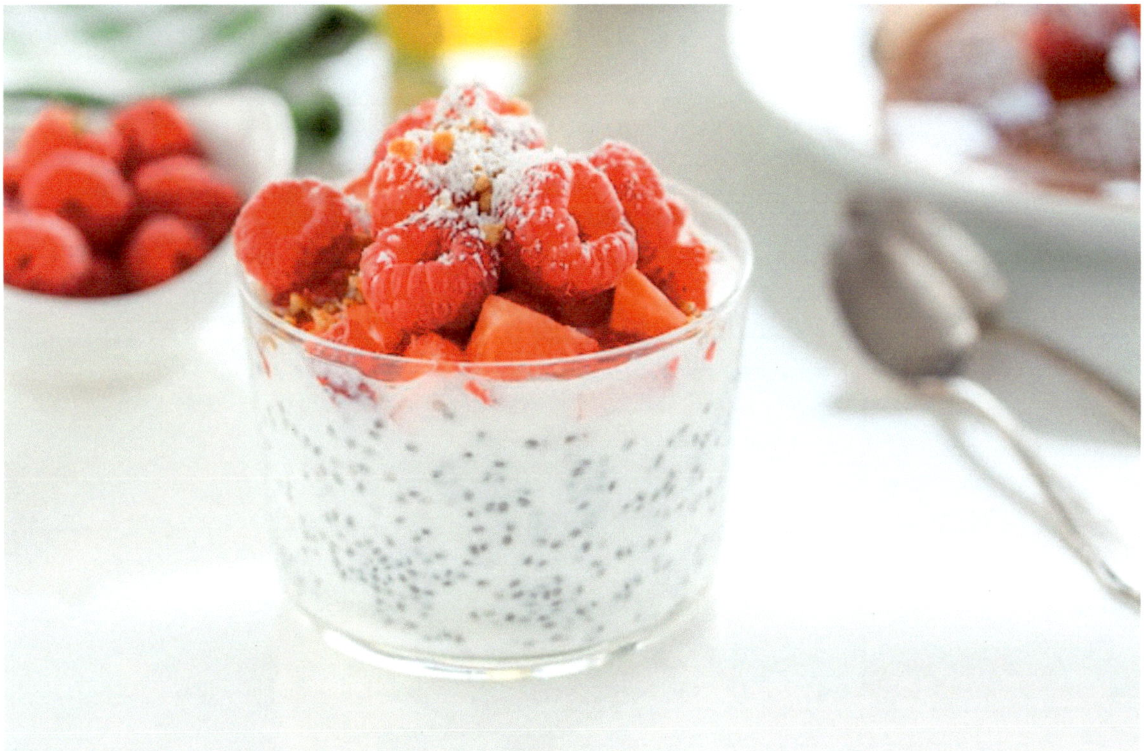

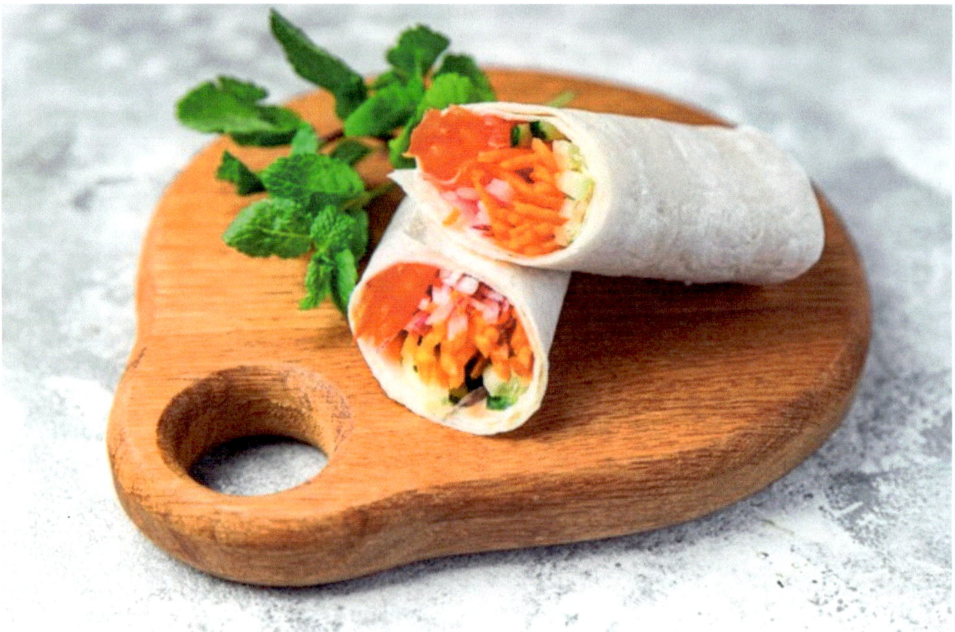

59. Turkey and Veggie Breakfast Burrito

Prep.Time: 10 min

Cook Time: 10 min

Serving: 1

Beverage pairing: Black Coffee

Ingredients:

- 1 whole wheat tortilla
- 2 large eggs, scrambled
- 2 slices turkey bacon, cooked and crumbled
- 1/4 cup diced bell peppers (any color)
- 1/4 cup diced onions
- 1/4 cup diced tomatoes
- 1/4 cup baby spinach leaves
- 1/4 cup shredded cheddar cheese (reduced-fat)
- Salt and pepper to taste

Preparation:

1. Heat a skillet over medium heat and lightly coat with cooking spray.
2. Add diced bell peppers and diced onions to the skillet. Cook until softened, about 5 minutes.
3. Add diced tomatoes and baby spinach leaves to the skillet. Cook until the spinach wilts, about 2 minutes.
4. In the center of the whole wheat tortilla, layer scrambled eggs, crumbled turkey bacon, cooked vegetables, and shredded cheddar cheese.
5. Season with salt and pepper to taste.
6. Fold in the sides of the tortilla and roll it up tightly to form a burrito.

Nutritional Facts (per serving):

- Calories: 300
- Carbohydrates: 20g
- Fat: 15g
- Protein: 20g

60. Greek Yogurt and Berry Smoothie

Prep.Time: 5 min	**Cook Time:** 0 min	**Serving:** 1	**Beverage pairing:** Herbal Tea

Ingredients:

- 1/2 cup Greek yogurt (unsweetened)
- 1/2 cup mixed berries (such as strawberries, blueberries, raspberries)
- 1/2 banana
- 1/2 cup unsweetened almond milk
- 1 tablespoon honey or maple syrup (optional)

Preparation:

1. In a blender, combine Greek yogurt, mixed berries, banana, almond milk, and honey or maple syrup (if using).
2. Blend until smooth and creamy.
3. Pour into a glass and serve immediately.

Nutrient Facts (per serving):

- Calories: 200
- Carbohydrates: 30g
- Fat: 3g
- Protein: 15g

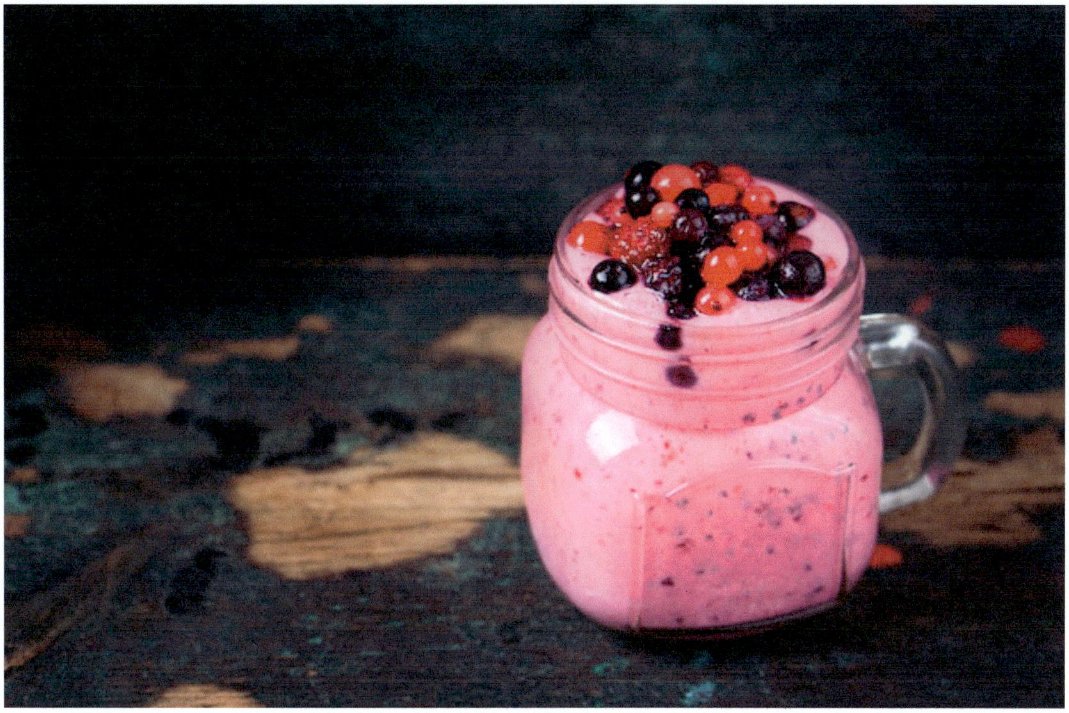

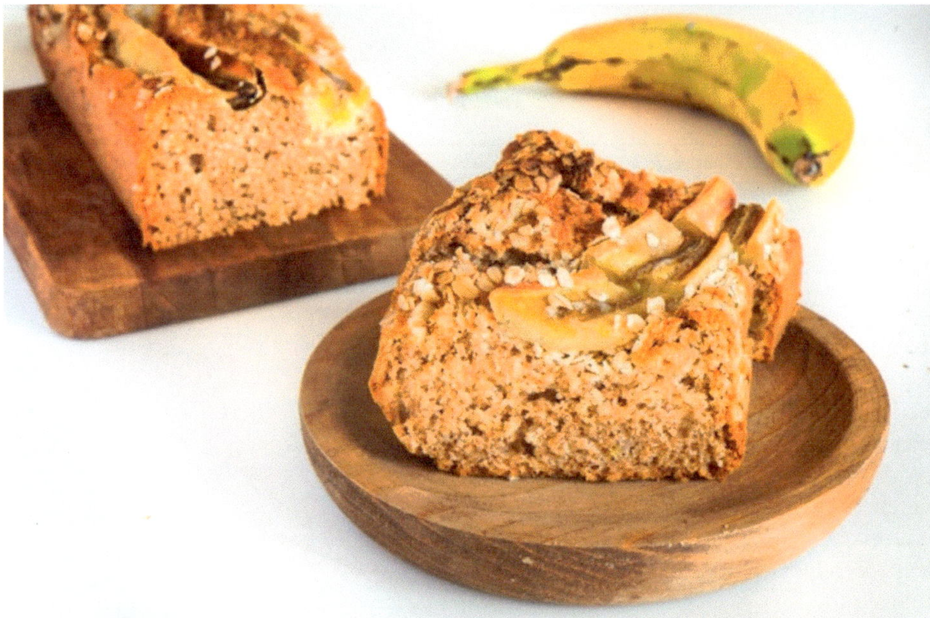

61. Almond Flour Banana Bread

Prep.Time: 10 min	Cook Time: 45-50 min	Serving: 10	Beverage pairing: Black Coffee

Ingredients:

- 2 ripe bananas, mashed
- 2 large eggs
- 1/4 cup honey or maple syrup
- 1/4 cup unsweetened applesauce
- 1 teaspoon vanilla extract
- 2 cups almond flour
- 1 teaspoon baking powder
- 1/2 teaspoon baking soda
- 1/4 teaspoon salt
- 1/2 teaspoon ground cinnamon
- 1/4 cup chopped walnuts (optional)

Preparation:

1. Preheat the oven to 350°F (175°C) and grease a loaf pan with cooking spray.
2. In a large bowl, whisk together mashed bananas, eggs, honey or maple syrup, unsweetened applesauce, and vanilla extract until well combined.
3. In another bowl, combine almond flour, baking powder, baking soda, salt, and ground cinnamon.
4. Gradually add the dry ingredients to the wet ingredients, stirring until just combined.
5. Fold in chopped walnuts if desired.
6. Pour the batter into the prepared loaf pan and spread it out evenly.
7. Bake for 45-50 minutes or until a toothpick inserted into the center comes out clean.
8. Allow the banana bread to cool in the pan for 10 minutes before transferring it to a wire rack to cool completely.

Nutritional Facts (1 slice-per serving):

- Calories: 200
- Carbohydrates: 20g
- Fat: 12g
- Protein: 6g

62. Spinach and Tomato Breakfast Pizza

Prep.Time:	Cook Time:	Serving:	Beverage pairing:
5 min	10-12 min	1	Herbal Tea

Ingredients:

- 1 whole wheat pita bread
- 2 tablespoons pizza sauce (no sugar added)
- 1/4 cup shredded mozzarella cheese (reduced-fat)
- 1/4 cup baby spinach leaves
- 1/4 cup diced tomatoes
- 2 large eggs
- Salt and pepper to taste
- Cooking spray

Preparation:

1. Preheat the oven to 375°F (190°C).
2. Place the whole wheat pita bread on a baking sheet lined with parchment paper.
3. Spread pizza sauce evenly over the pita bread.
4. Sprinkle shredded mozzarella cheese over the sauce.
5. Top with baby spinach leaves and diced tomatoes.
6. Create two small wells in the toppings and crack one egg into each well.
7. Season with salt and pepper to taste.
8. Bake for 10-12 minutes or until the egg whites are set and the yolks are still runny.
9. Remove from the oven and let it cool for a few minutes before slicing and serving.

Nutrient Facts (per serving):

- Calories: 250
- Carbohydrates: 20g
- Fat: 10g
- Protein: 15g

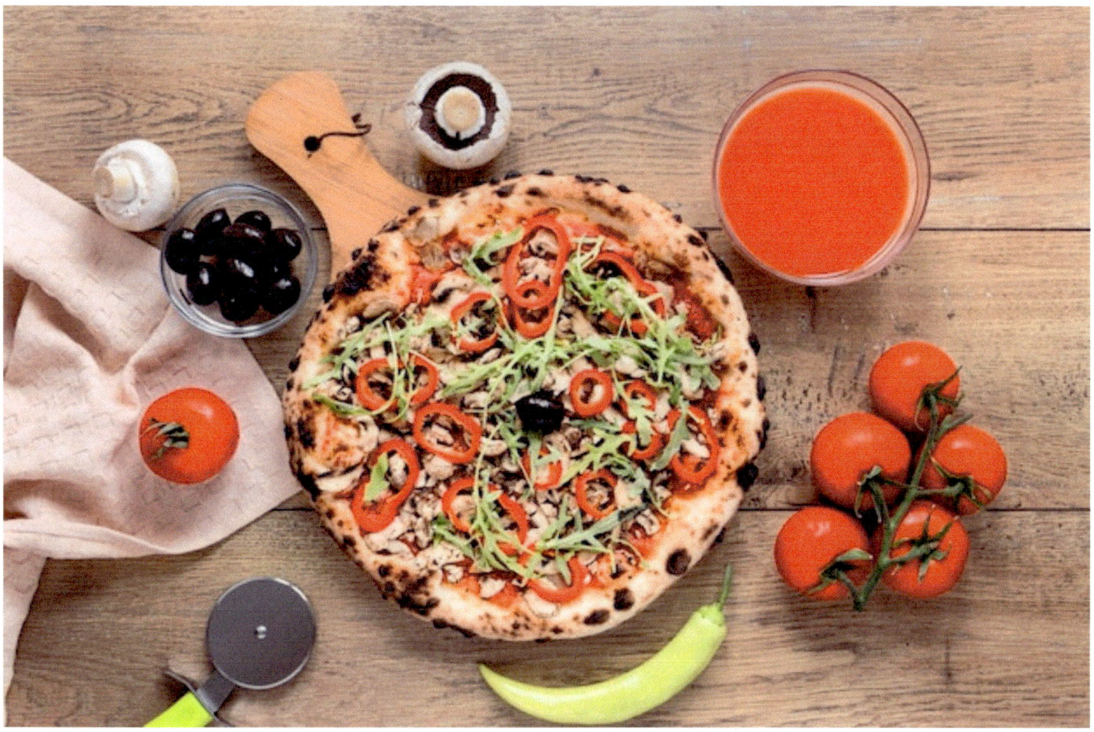

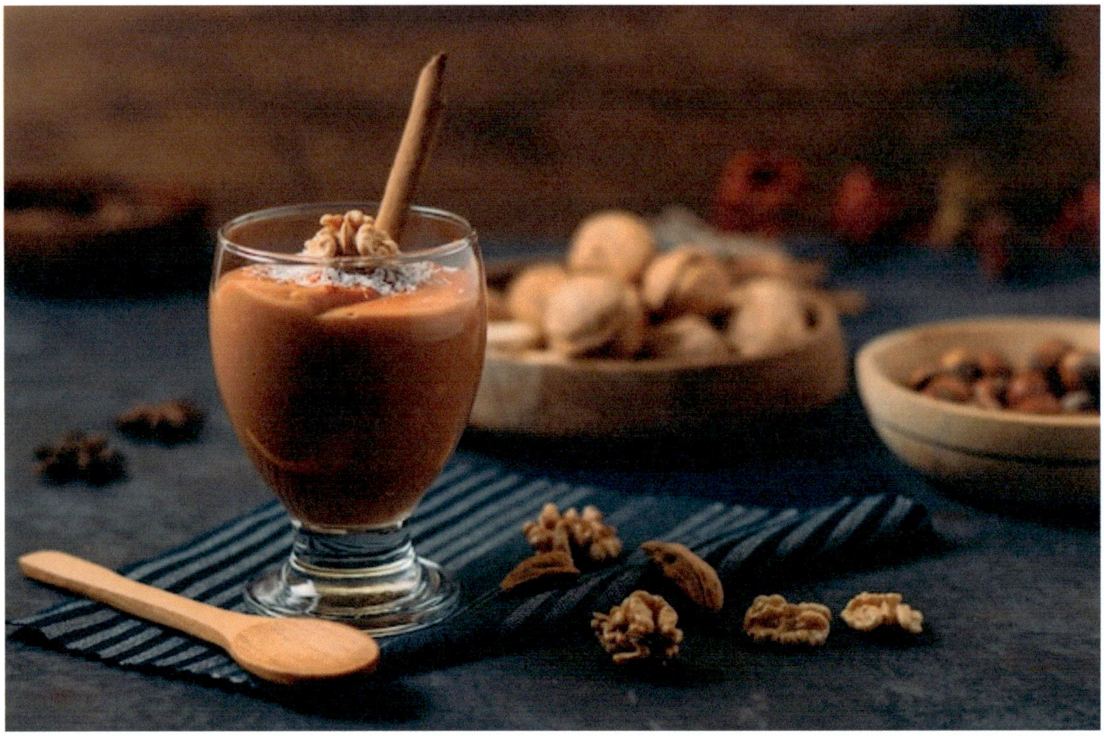

63. Hazelnut Mocha Protein Smoothie

Prep.Time: 5 min | **Cook Time:** 0 min | **Serving:** 1 | **Beverage pairing:** Almond Milk

Ingredients:

- 1 ripe banana
- 1 tablespoon cocoa powder
- 1 tablespoon hazelnut butter
- 1/2 cup brewed coffee, chilled
- 1/2 cup unsweetened almond milk
- 1 scoop chocolate protein powder
- Ice cubes (optional)
- Whipped cream for topping (optional)
- Crushed hazelnuts for garnish (optional)

Preparation:

1. In a blender, combine ripe banana, cocoa powder, hazelnut butter, brewed coffee, almond milk, and chocolate protein powder.
2. Blend until smooth and creamy.
3. If desired, add ice cubes for a colder and thicker texture and blend again.
4. Pour into a glass, and top with whipped cream and crushed hazelnuts if desired.
5. Serve immediately.

Nutritional Facts (per serving):

- Calories: 250
- Carbohydrates: 30g
- Fat: 8g
- Protein: 18g

64. Quinoa and Kale Breakfast Bowl

Prep.Time:	Cook Time:	Serving:	Beverage pairing:
15 min	15 min	1	Herbal Tea

Ingredients:

- 1/2 cup cooked quinoa
- 1 cup chopped kale
- 1/4 cup diced tomatoes
- 1/4 cup diced bell peppers (any color)
- 1/4 cup diced onions
- 2 large eggs
- 1 tablespoon olive oil
- Salt and pepper to taste
- Optional toppings: sliced avocado, crumbled feta cheese, hot sauce

Preparation:

1. Heat olive oil in a skillet over medium heat.
2. Add diced onions and diced bell peppers to the skillet. Cook until softened, about 5 minutes.
3. Add chopped kale and diced tomatoes to the skillet. Cook until the kale wilts, about 2-3 minutes.
4. Push the vegetables to one side of the skillet and crack the eggs into the empty space.
5. Cook the eggs to your desired doneness, either scrambled or sunny-side-up.
6. Season the vegetables and eggs with salt and pepper to taste.
7. In a bowl, layer cooked quinoa with the sautéed vegetables and eggs.
8. Serve hot with optional toppings such as sliced avocado, crumbled feta cheese, or hot sauce.

Nutrient Facts (per serving):

- Calories: 350
- Carbohydrates: 30g
- Fat: 18g
- Protein: 18g

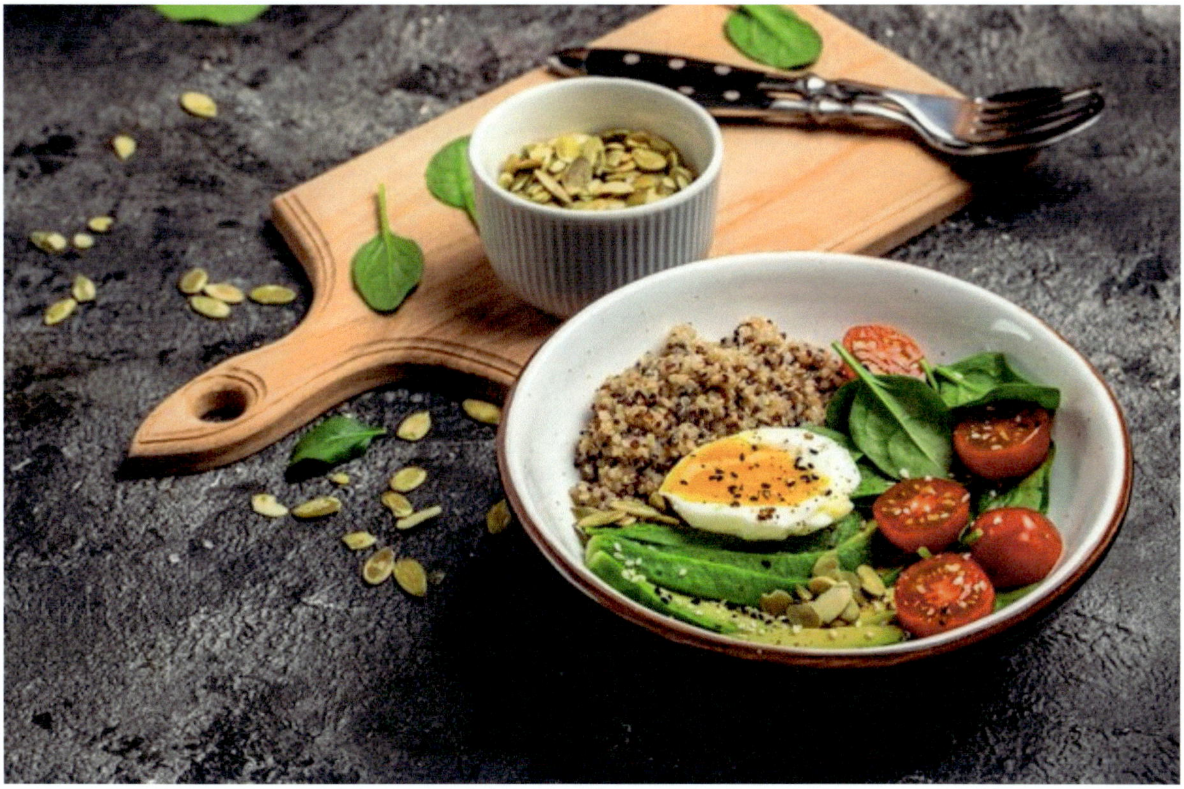

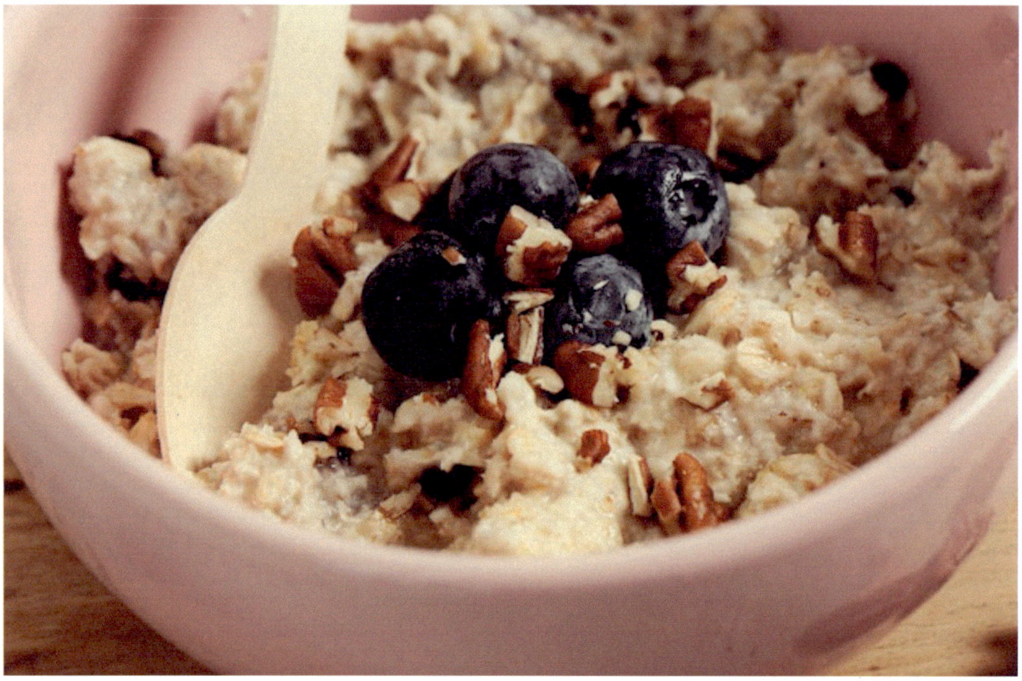

65. Blackberry Walnut Overnight Oats

Prep.Time:	Cook Time:	Serving:	Beverage pairing:
5 min	0 min	1	Black Coffee

Ingredients:

- 1/2 cup rolled oats
- 1/2 cup unsweetened almond milk
- 1/4 cup blackberries
- 2 tablespoons chopped walnuts
- 1 tablespoon honey or maple syrup (optional)

Preparation:

1. In a jar or container, combine rolled oats and unsweetened almond milk.
2. Add blackberries and chopped walnuts on top.
3. Drizzle with honey or maple syrup if desired.
4. Stir well to combine all ingredients.
5. Cover the jar/container and refrigerate overnight or for at least 4 hours.
6. In the morning, give the oats a stir and enjoy cold.

Nutritional Facts (per serving):

- Calories: 250
- Carbohydrates: 30g
- Fat: 10g
- Protein: 7g

66. Asparagus and Goat Cheese Frittata

Prep.Time:	Cook Time:	Serving:	Beverage pairing:
10 min	20 min	2	Black Coffee

Ingredients:

- 4 large eggs
- 1/4 cup milk (any type)
- 1/2 cup chopped asparagus
- 1/4 cup crumbled goat cheese
- 1/4 cup diced onions
- 1 tablespoon olive oil
- Salt and pepper to taste

Preparation:

1. Preheat the oven to 350°F (175°C).
2. In a bowl, whisk together eggs and milk until well combined. Season with salt and pepper.
3. Heat olive oil in an oven-safe skillet over medium heat.
4. Add diced onions and chopped asparagus to the skillet. Cook until the vegetables are tender, about 5 minutes.
5. Pour the egg mixture over the cooked vegetables in the skillet.
6. Sprinkle crumbled goat cheese evenly over the top.
7. Transfer the skillet to the preheated oven and bake for 12-15 minutes or until the frittata is set and the edges are golden brown.
8. Remove from the oven and let it cool for a few minutes before slicing and serving.

Nutrient Facts (per serving):

- Calories: 250
- Carbohydrates: 5g
- Fat: 18g
- Protein: 15g

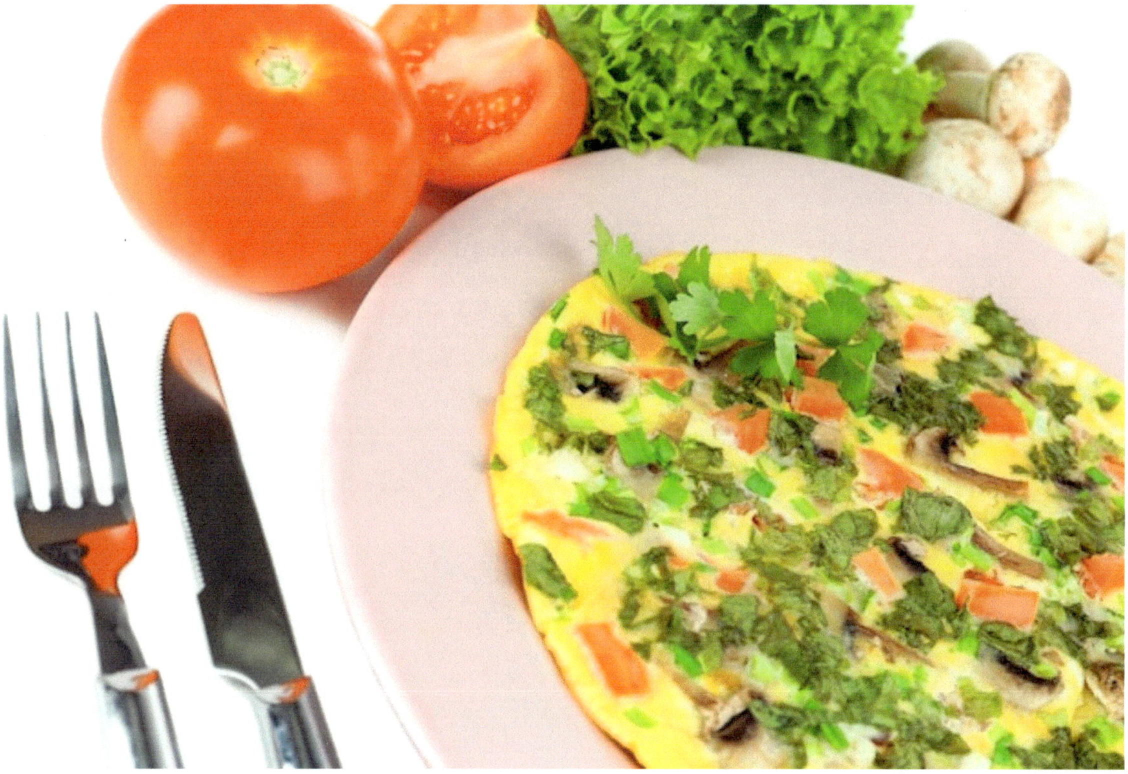

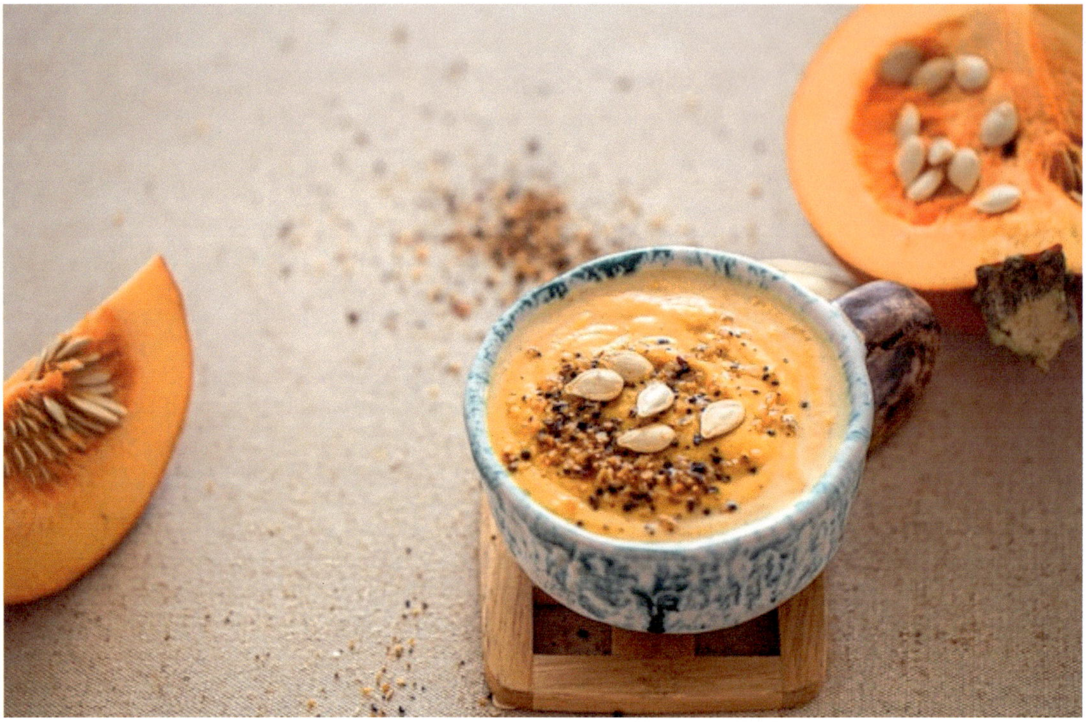

67. Pumpkin Spice Chia Seed Pudding

Prep.Time:	Cook Time:	Serving:	Beverage pairing:
5 min	0 min	1	Black Coffee

Ingredients:

- 2 tablespoons chia seeds
- 1/2 cup unsweetened almond milk
- 1/4 cup pumpkin puree
- 1 tablespoon maple syrup
- 1/2 teaspoon pumpkin pie spice
- Optional toppings: chopped pecans, cinnamon

Preparation:

1. In a bowl, mix together chia seeds, almond milk, pumpkin puree, maple syrup, and pumpkin pie spice until well combined.
2. Cover the bowl and refrigerate for at least 2 hours or overnight, allowing the chia seeds to gel and thicken.
3. Before serving, stir the pudding well and top with chopped pecans and a sprinkle of cinnamon if desired.

Nutritional Facts (per serving):

- Calories: 200
- Carbohydrates: 20g
- Fat: 10g
- Protein: 6g

68. Banana Walnut Breakfast Cookies

Prep.Time: 10 min

Cook Time: 12-15 min

Serving: 4

Beverage pairing: Herbal Tea

Ingredients:

- 1 ripe banana, mashed
- 1 cup rolled oats
- 1/4 cup chopped walnuts
- 2 tablespoons unsweetened almond milk
- 1 tablespoon honey or maple syrup
- 1/2 teaspoon vanilla extract
- Pinch of cinnamon
- Pinch of salt

Preparation:

1. Preheat the oven to 350°F (175°C) and line a baking sheet with parchment paper.
2. In a bowl, combine mashed banana, rolled oats, chopped walnuts, almond milk, honey or maple syrup, vanilla extract, cinnamon, and salt. Mix well.
3. Scoop out spoonfuls of the mixture and place them onto the prepared baking sheet, flattening them slightly with the back of a spoon.
4. Bake for 12-15 minutes or until the cookies are golden brown and set.
5. Allow the cookies to cool on the baking sheet for a few minutes before transferring them to a wire rack to cool completely.

Nutritional Facts (per serving - 2 cookies):

- Calories: 200
- Carbohydrates: 25g
- Fat: 8g
- Protein: 5g

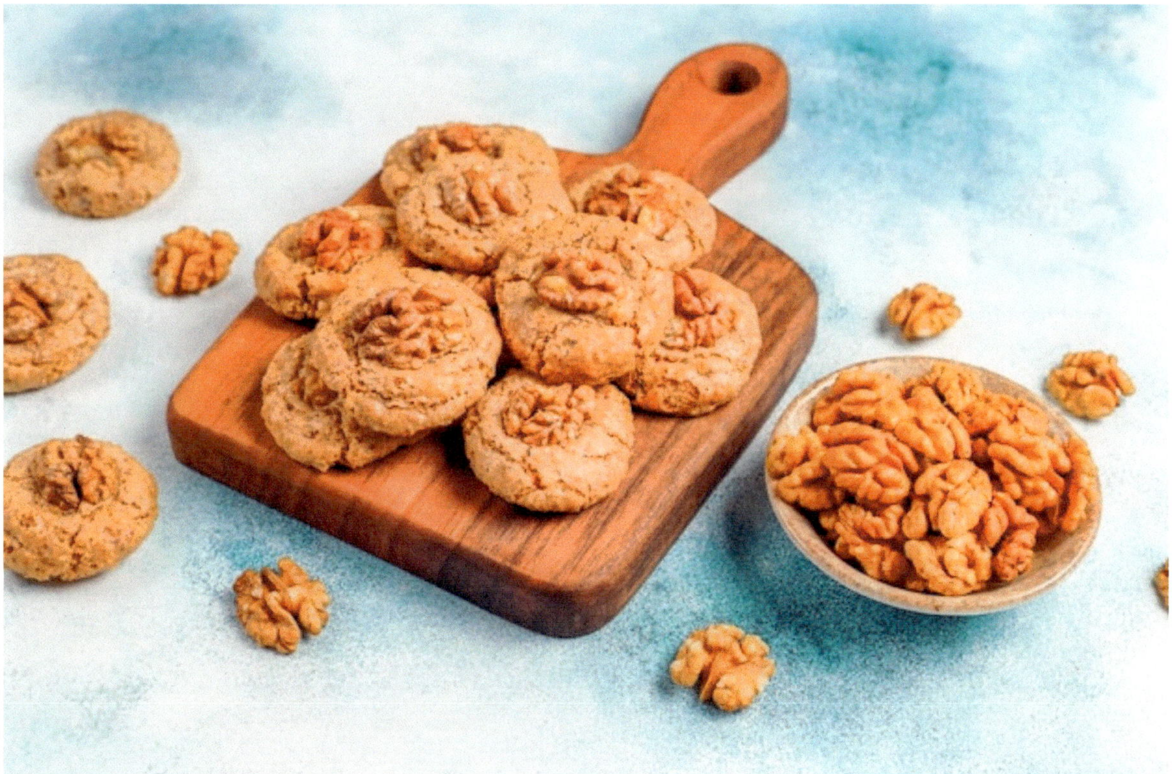

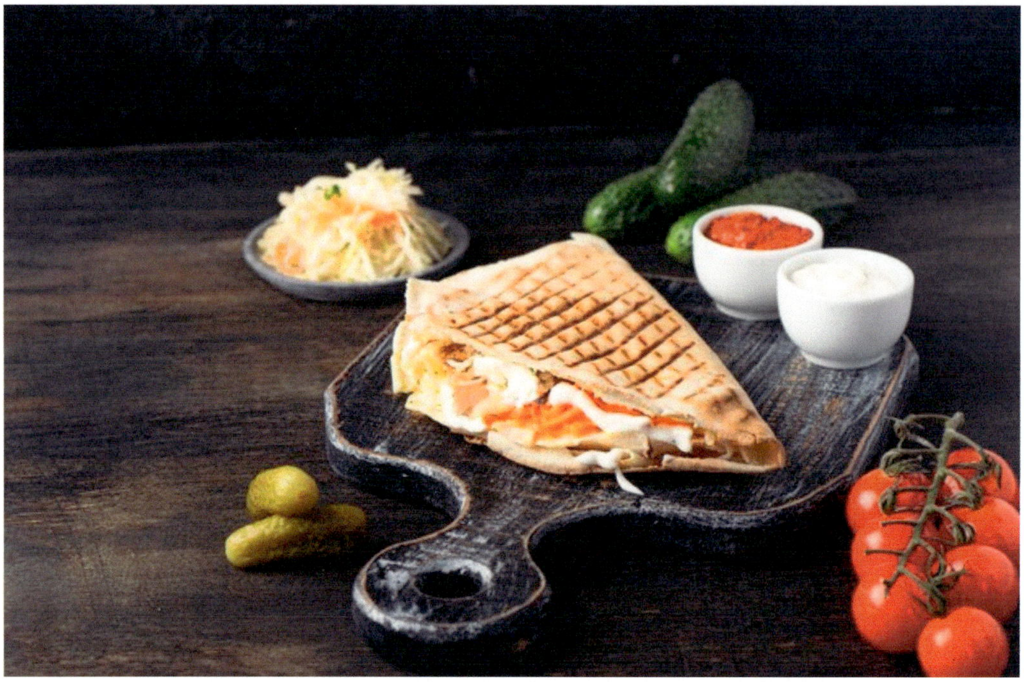

69. Mediterranean Breakfast Panini

Prep.Time:	Cook Time:	Serving:	Beverage pairing:
10 min	10 min	1	Black Coffee

Ingredients:

- 2 slices whole grain bread
- 2 large eggs
- 2 slices turkey breast
- 1/4 cup sliced tomatoes
- 1/4 cup baby spinach leaves
- 2 tablespoons crumbled feta cheese
- 1 tablespoon olive oil
- Salt and pepper to taste

Preparation:

1. Preheat a panini press or grill pan over medium heat.
2. In a bowl, beat the eggs and season with salt and pepper.
3. Heat olive oil in a skillet over medium heat. Pour in the beaten eggs and cook until set, then fold in half to form an omelette.
4. Assemble the panini: Place one slice of whole grain bread on a flat surface. Layer turkey breast, sliced tomatoes, baby spinach leaves, the cooked omelette, and crumbled feta cheese. Top with the other slice of bread.
5. Place the assembled panini in the panini press or grill pan. Cook for 3-5 minutes, or until the bread is golden brown and crispy, and the filling is warmed through.
6. Remove from heat, slice in half if desired, and serve hot.

Nutritional Facts (per serving):

- Calories: 350
- Carbohydrates: 25g
- Fat: 18g
- Protein: 22g

70. Strawberry Cheesecake Parfait

Prep.Time: 5 min	**Cook Time:** 0 min	**Serving:** 1	**Beverage pairing:** Herbal Tea

Ingredients:

- 1/2 cup Greek yogurt (unsweetened)
- 1/4 cup diced strawberries
- 2 tablespoons crushed graham crackers
- 1 tablespoon honey or maple syrup (optional)
- Fresh mint leaves for garnish (optional)

Preparation:

1. In a glass or parfait dish, layer Greek yogurt, diced strawberries, and crushed graham crackers.
2. Repeat the layers until the glass is filled, ending with a layer of crushed graham crackers on top.
3. Drizzle with honey or maple syrup if desired.
4. Garnish with fresh mint leaves if desired.
5. Serve immediately or refrigerate until ready to serve.

Nutritional Facts (per serving):

- Calories: 200
- Carbohydrates: 25g
- Fat: 5g
- Protein: 15g

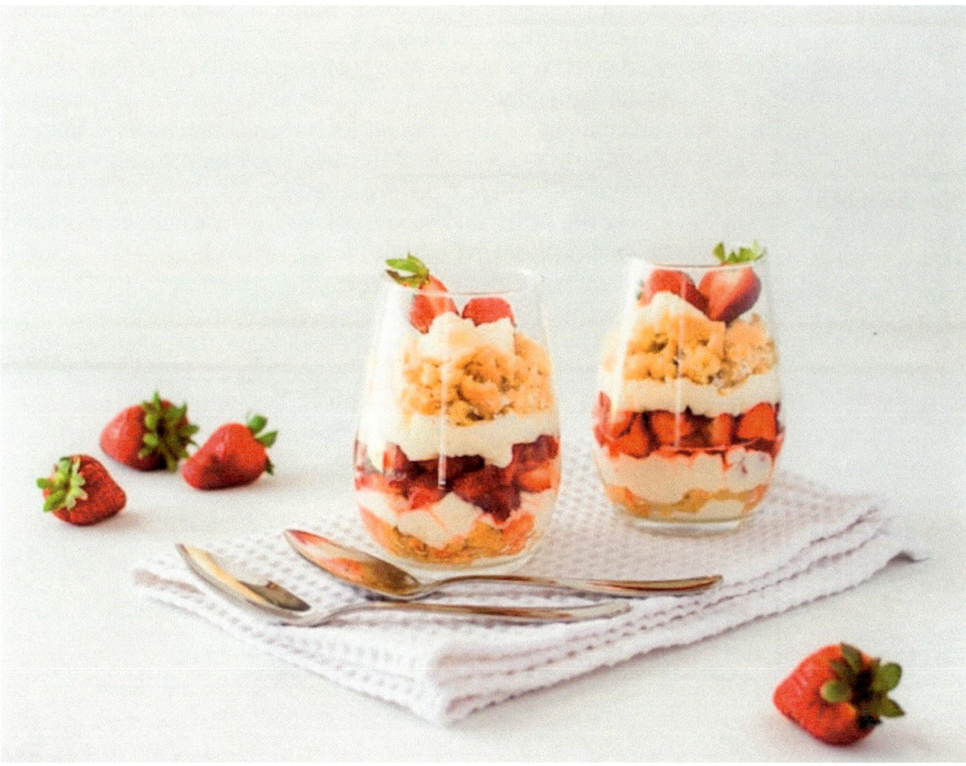

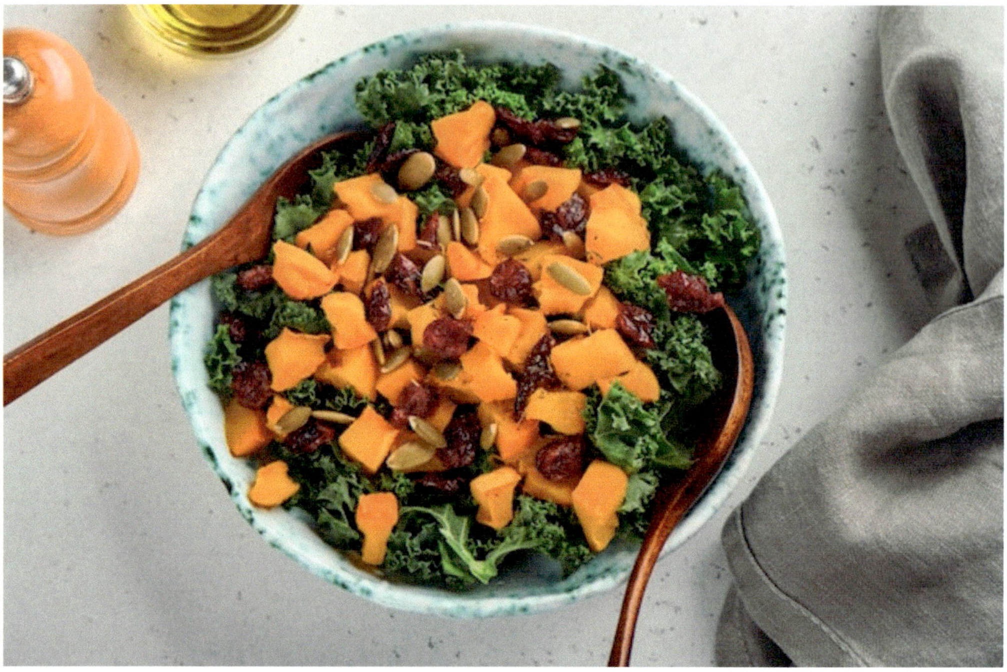

71. Sweet Potato and Kale Breakfast Skillet

Prep.Time:	Cook Time:	Serving:	Beverage pairing:
10 min	20 min	1	Black Coffee

Ingredients:

- 1 small sweet potato, peeled and diced
- 1 cup chopped kale
- 2 eggs
- 1/4 cup diced onions
- 1/4 cup diced bell peppers (any color)
- 1 tablespoon olive oil
- Salt and pepper to taste

Preparation:

1. Heat olive oil in a skillet over medium heat.
2. Add diced sweet potato to the skillet and cook until softened, about 8-10 minutes, stirring occasionally.
3. Add diced onions and diced bell peppers to the skillet. Cook until softened, about 5 minutes.
4. Add chopped kale to the skillet and cook until wilted, about 2-3 minutes.
5. Create two wells in the skillet and crack one egg into each well.
6. Season with salt and pepper to taste.
7. Cover the skillet and cook until the eggs are cooked to your desired doneness, about 5-7 minutes for runny yolks.
8. Remove from heat and serve hot.

Nutritional Facts (per serving):

- Calories: 300
- Carbohydrates: 25g
- Fat: 15g
- Protein: 12g

72. Chocolate Peanut Butter Protein Pancakes

Prep.Time: 10 min

Cook Time: 10 min

Serving: 1

Beverage pairing: Herbal Tea

Ingredients:

- 1/2 cup rolled oats
- 1/2 banana
- 1 scoop chocolate protein powder
- 1 tablespoon peanut butter (unsweetened)
- 1/4 cup unsweetened almond milk
- 1/2 teaspoon baking powder
- Cooking spray

Preparation:

1. In a blender, combine rolled oats, banana, chocolate protein powder, peanut butter, unsweetened almond milk, and baking powder. Blend until smooth.
2. Heat a non-stick skillet over medium heat and lightly coat with cooking spray.
3. Pour the pancake batter onto the skillet to form pancakes of desired size.
4. Cook until bubbles form on the surface of the pancakes, then flip and cook until golden brown on both sides.
5. Repeat with the remaining batter.
6. Serve hot with toppings of your choice such as sliced bananas, chopped nuts, or a drizzle of peanut butter.

Nutritional Facts (per serving):

- Calories: 350
- Carbohydrates: 30g
- Fat: 12g
- Protein: 25g

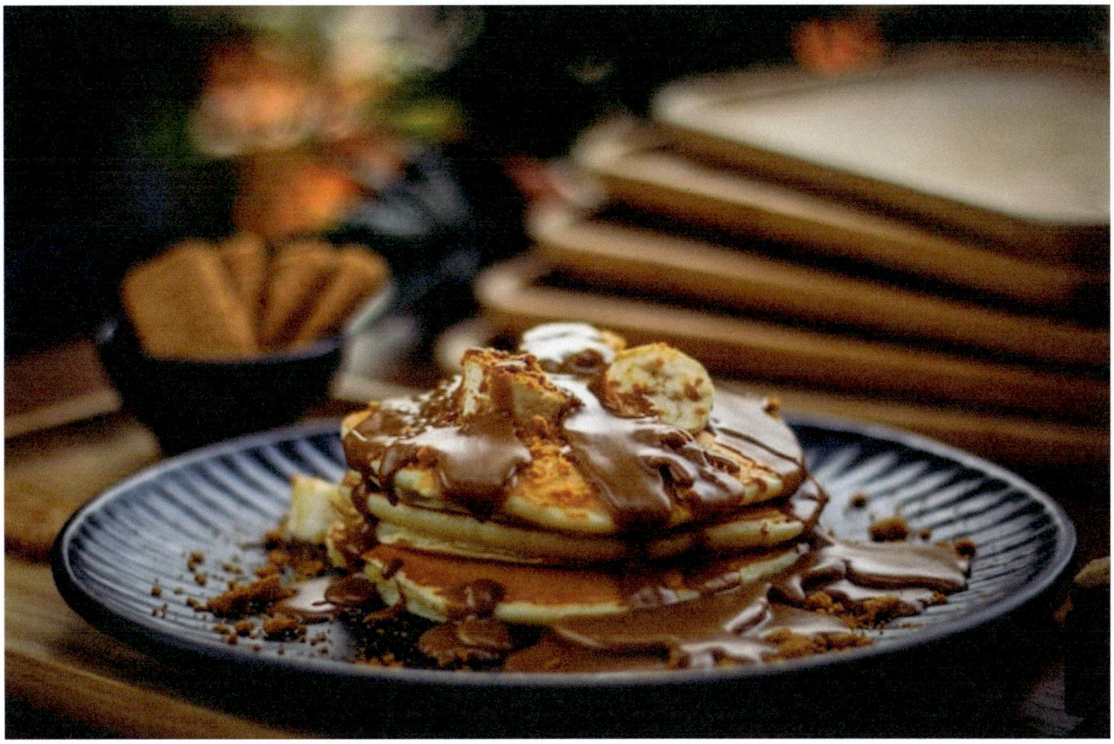

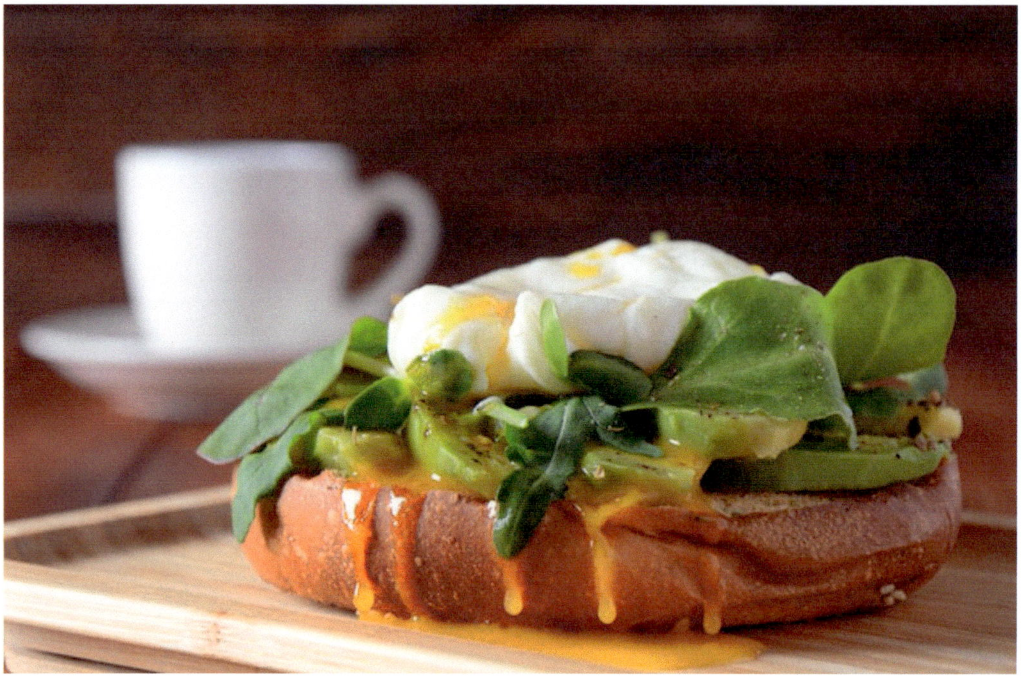

73. Egg and Spinach Breakfast Sandwich

Prep.Time:	Cook Time:	Serving:	Beverage pairing:
5 min	5 min	1	Black Coffee

Ingredients:

- 1 whole wheat English muffin, split and toasted
- 1 large egg
- 1/4 cup baby spinach leaves
- 1 slice tomato
- 1 slice reduced-fat cheddar cheese
- Salt and pepper to taste
- Cooking spray

Preparation:

1. Heat a skillet over medium heat and lightly coat with cooking spray.
2. Crack the egg into the skillet and cook until the whites are set, about 2-3 minutes.
3. Season with salt and pepper to taste.
4. Assemble the sandwich: Place the cooked egg on the bottom half of the toasted English muffin. Top with baby spinach leaves, tomato slice, and cheddar cheese. Cover with the top half of the English muffin.
5. Serve hot.

Nutritional Facts (per serving):

- Calories: 300
- Carbohydrates: 25g
- Fat: 12g
- Protein: 20g

74. Cinnamon Apple Quinoa Bowl

Prep.Time:	Cook Time:	Serving:	Beverage pairing:
5 min	0 min	1	Herbal Tea

Ingredients:

- 1/2 cup cooked quinoa
- 1/2 apple, diced
- 1 tablespoon chopped walnuts
- 1 tablespoon raisins
- 1/2 teaspoon ground cinnamon
- 1 teaspoon honey or maple syrup (optional)
- 1/4 cup unsweetened almond milk

Preparation:

1. In a bowl, combine cooked quinoa, diced apple, chopped walnuts, raisins, and ground cinnamon.
2. Drizzle with honey or maple syrup if desired.
3. Pour unsweetened almond milk over the quinoa mixture.
4. Stir well to combine all ingredients.
5. Microwave for 1-2 minutes until warm, or enjoy cold.

Nutritional Facts (per serving):

- Calories: 250
- Carbohydrates: 35g
- Fat: 8g
- Protein: 7g

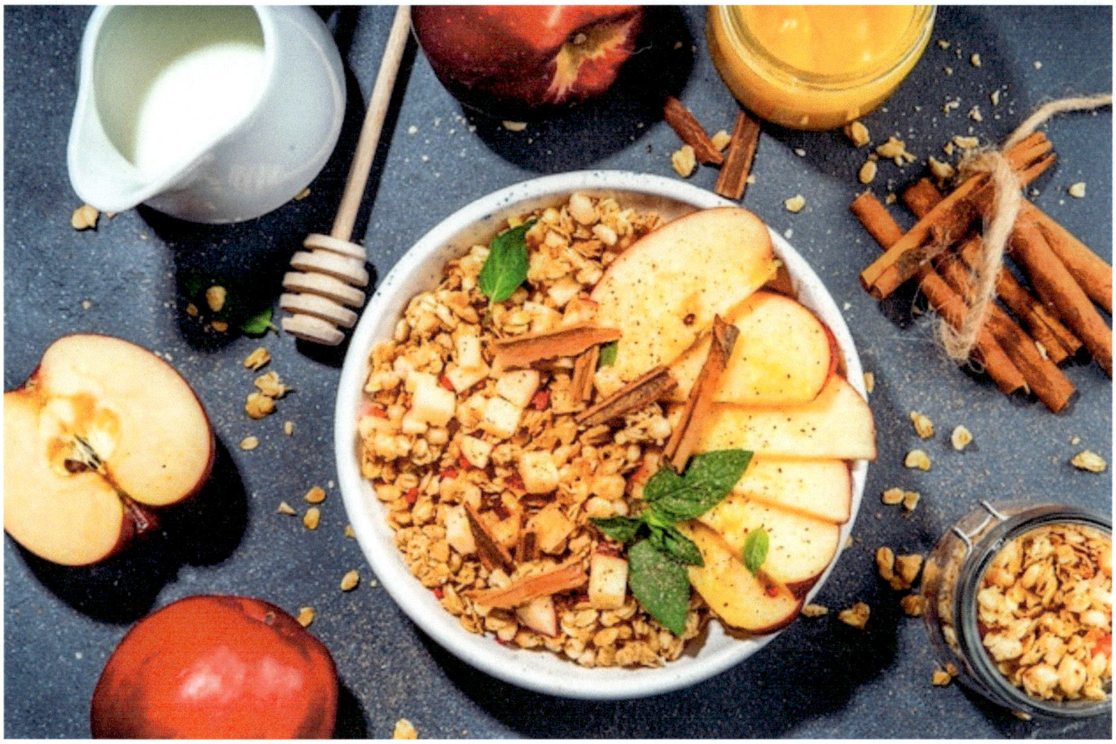

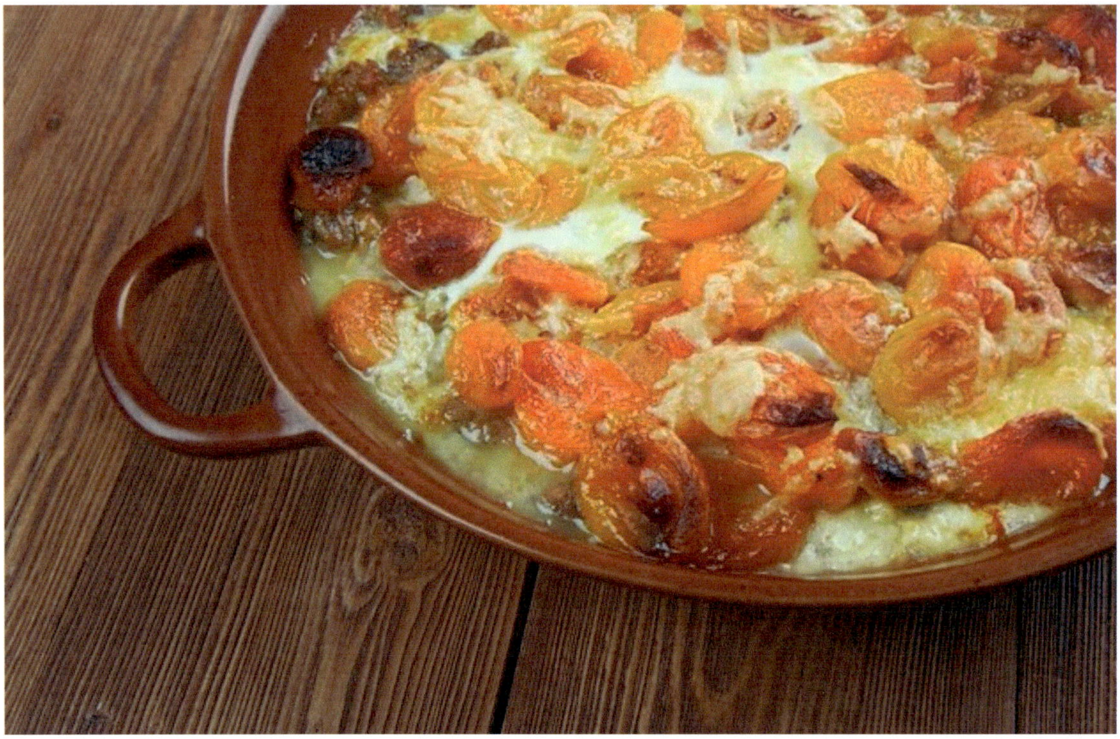

75. Southwest Breakfast Casserole

Prep.Time: 15 min

Cook Time: 25-30 min

Serving: 6

Beverage pairing: Black Coffee

Ingredients:

- 6 large eggs
- 1/2 cup milk (any type)
- 1 cup cooked quinoa
- 1 cup black beans, drained and rinsed
- 1 cup diced bell peppers (any color)
- 1 cup diced tomatoes
- 1/2 cup diced onions
- 1 cup shredded cheddar cheese (reduced-fat)
- 1 teaspoon chili powder
- 1/2 teaspoon ground cumin
- Salt and pepper to taste

Preparation:

1. Preheat the oven to 375°F (190°C). Lightly grease a baking dish with cooking spray.
2. In a large mixing bowl, whisk together eggs, milk, chili powder, ground cumin, salt, and pepper.
3. Stir in cooked quinoa, black beans, diced bell peppers, diced tomatoes, diced onions, and shredded cheddar cheese until well combined.
4. Pour the mixture into the prepared baking dish and spread it out evenly.
5. Bake in the preheated oven for 25-30 minutes or until the eggs are set and the top is golden brown.
6. Remove from the oven and let it cool for a few minutes before slicing and serving.

Nutritional Facts (per serving):

- Calories: 300
- Carbohydrates: 20g
- Fat: 15g
- Protein: 20g

76. Blueberry Almond Butter Smoothie

Prep.Time: 5 min

Cook Time: 0 min

Serving: 1

Beverage pairing: Almond Milk

Ingredients:

- 1/2 cup frozen blueberries
- 1 tablespoon almond butter (unsweetened)
- 1/2 cup Greek yogurt (unsweetened)
- 1/2 cup unsweetened almond milk
- 1 tablespoon honey or maple syrup (optional)
- Ice cubes (optional)

Preparation:

1. In a blender, combine frozen blueberries, almond butter, Greek yogurt, almond milk, and honey or maple syrup (if using).
2. If desired, add ice cubes for a colder and thicker texture.
3. Blend until smooth and creamy.
4. Pour into a glass and serve immediately.

Nutritional Facts (per serving):

- Calories: 200
- Carbohydrates: 20g
- Fat: 8g
- Protein: 12g

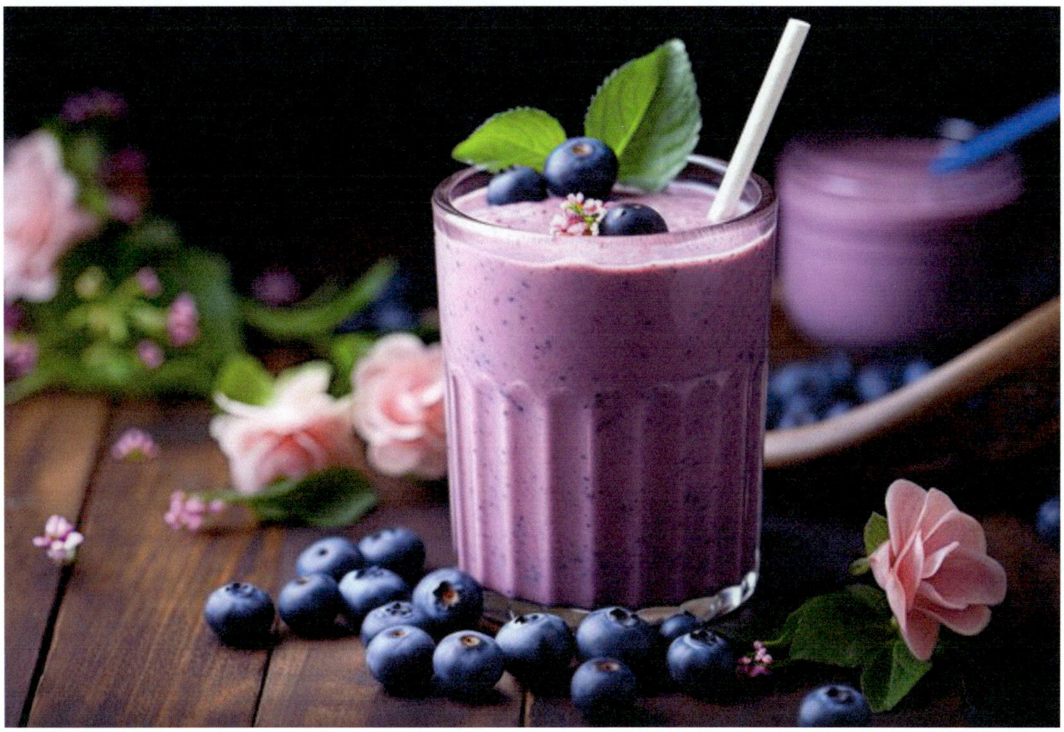

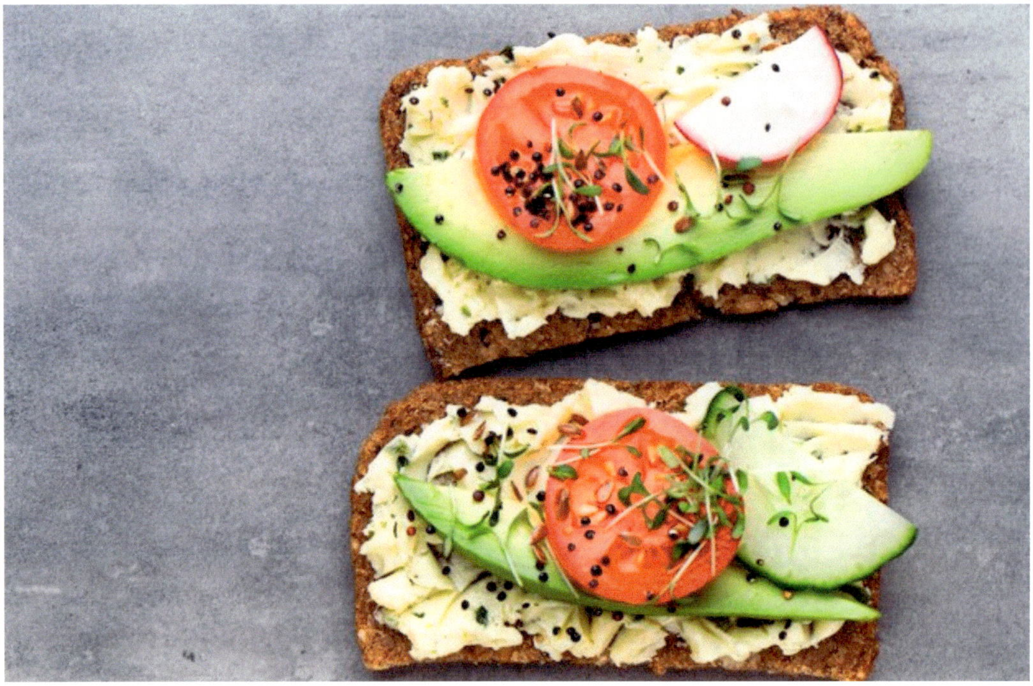

77. Tomato Basil Avocado Toast

Prep.Time: 15 min	**Cook Time:** 0 min	**Serving:** 1	**Beverage pairing:** Black Coffee

Ingredients:

- 2 slices whole grain bread, toasted
- 1/2 avocado, mashed
- 1 small tomato, sliced
- Fresh basil leaves
- Salt and pepper to taste

Preparation:

1. Spread mashed avocado evenly onto the toasted whole grain bread slices.
2. Top with sliced tomatoes and fresh basil leaves.
3. Season with salt and pepper to taste.
4. Serve immediately.

Nutritional Facts (per serving):

- Calories: 250
- Carbohydrates: 25g
- Fat: 10g
- Protein: 8g

78. Pineapple Coconut Chia Pudding

Prep.Time:	Cook Time:	Serving:	Beverage pairing:
5 min	0 min	1	Herbal Tea

Ingredients:

- 2 tablespoons chia seeds
- 1/2 cup coconut milk
- 1/4 cup unsweetened pineapple chunks
- 1 tablespoon shredded coconut (unsweetened)
- 1 teaspoon honey or maple syrup (optional)

Preparation:

1. In a bowl, mix together chia seeds and coconut milk until well combined.
2. Gently fold in unsweetened pineapple chunks.
3. Cover the bowl and refrigerate for at least 2 hours or overnight, allowing the chia seeds to gel and thicken.
4. Before serving, sprinkle shredded coconut on top and drizzle with honey or maple syrup if desired.

Nutritional Facts (per serving):

- Calories: 200
- Carbohydrates: 20g
- Fat: 10g
- Protein: 6g

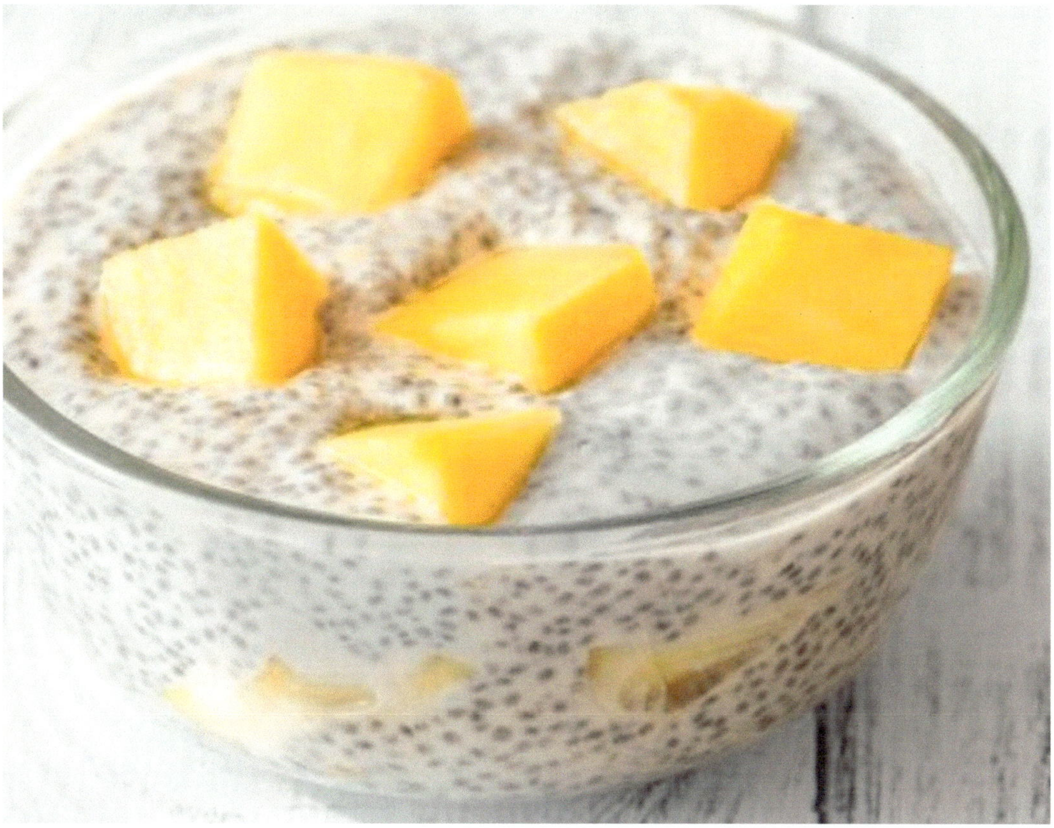

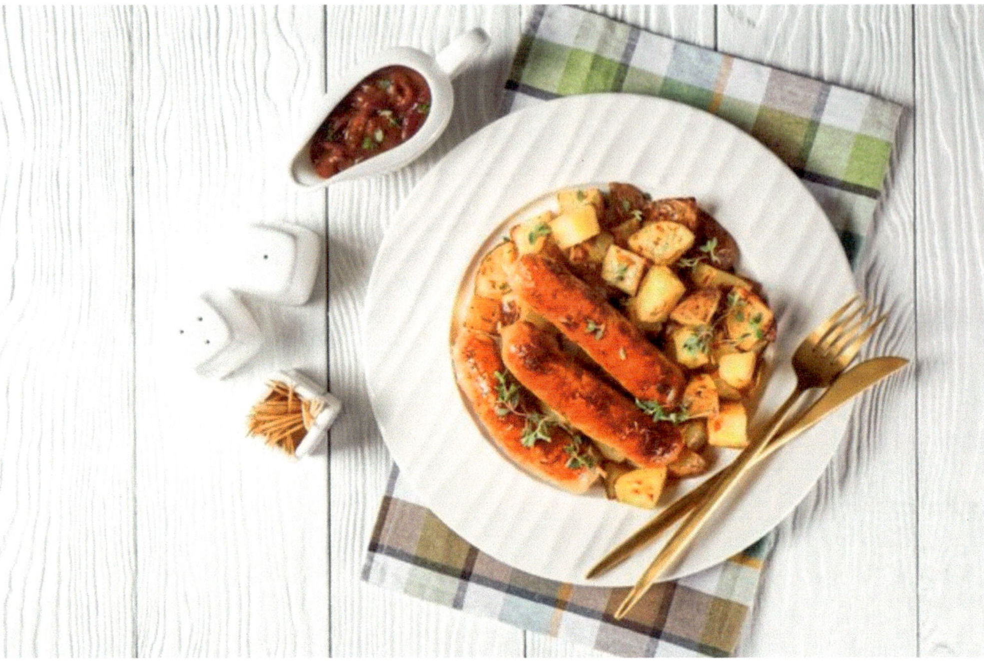

79. Turkey Sausage and Sweet Potato Hash

Prep.Time: 10 min

Cook Time: 20 min

Serving: 4

Beverage pairing: Black Coffee

Ingredients:

- 1/2 lb turkey sausage, casings removed
- 2 cups diced sweet potatoes
- 1/2 cup diced bell peppers (any color)
- 1/4 cup diced onions
- 2 cloves garlic, minced
- 1 teaspoon paprika
- 1/2 teaspoon dried thyme
- Salt and pepper to taste
- 2 tablespoons chopped fresh parsley (for garnish)
- Cooking spray

Preparation:

1. Heat a skillet over medium heat and lightly coat with cooking spray.
2. Add turkey sausage to the skillet and cook, breaking it apart with a spoon, until browned and cooked through.
3. Remove the cooked sausage from the skillet and set aside.
4. In the same skillet, add diced sweet potatoes. Cook until they start to soften, about 8-10 minutes, stirring occasionally.
5. Add diced bell peppers, diced onions, and minced garlic to the skillet. Cook until the vegetables are tender, about 5 minutes.
6. Return the cooked turkey sausage to the skillet. Sprinkle paprika, dried thyme, salt, and pepper over the mixture. Stir well to combine.
7. Cook for an additional 2-3 minutes to heat everything through.
8. Garnish with chopped fresh parsley before serving.

Nutritional Facts (per serving):

- Calories: 300
- Carbohydrates: 25g
- Fat: 15g
- Protein: 18g

80. Raspberry Chocolate Chip Muffins

Prep.Time:	Cook Time:	Serving:	Beverage pairing:
10 min	18-20 min	12	Herbal Tea

Ingredients:

- 1 cup whole wheat flour
- 1/2 cup rolled oats
- 1/4 cup unsweetened cocoa powder
- 1/4 cup honey or maple syrup
- 1/4 cup unsweetened applesauce
- 1/4 cup Greek yogurt (unsweetened)
- 1/4 cup unsweetened almond milk
- 1/4 cup dark chocolate chips
- 1/2 cup fresh raspberries
- 1 teaspoon baking powder

Preparation:

1. Preheat the oven to 350°F (175°C). Line a muffin tin with paper liners or grease with cooking spray.
2. In a large mixing bowl, whisk together whole wheat flour, rolled oats, cocoa powder, baking powder, baking soda, and salt.
3. In another bowl, beat the egg and mix in honey or maple syrup, unsweetened applesauce, Greek yogurt, unsweetened almond milk, and vanilla extract until well combined.
4. Pour the wet ingredients into the dry ingredients and mix until just combined.
5. Gently fold in dark chocolate chips and fresh raspberries.
6. Divide the batter evenly among the muffin cups, filling each about 3/4 full.
7. Bake in the preheated oven for 18-20 minutes or until a toothpick inserted into the center comes out clean.
8. Remove from the oven and let the muffins cool in the tin for a few minutes before transferring to a wire rack to cool completely

Nutritional Facts (per muffin):

- Calories: 180
- Carbohydrates: 25g
- Fat: 7g
- Protein: 5g

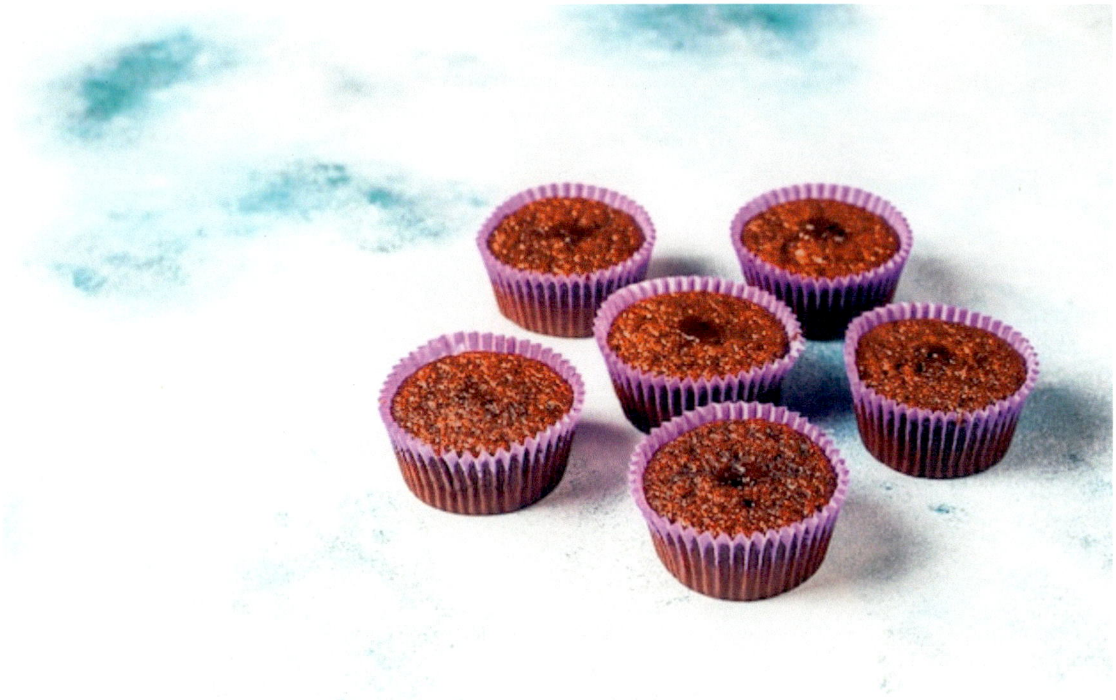

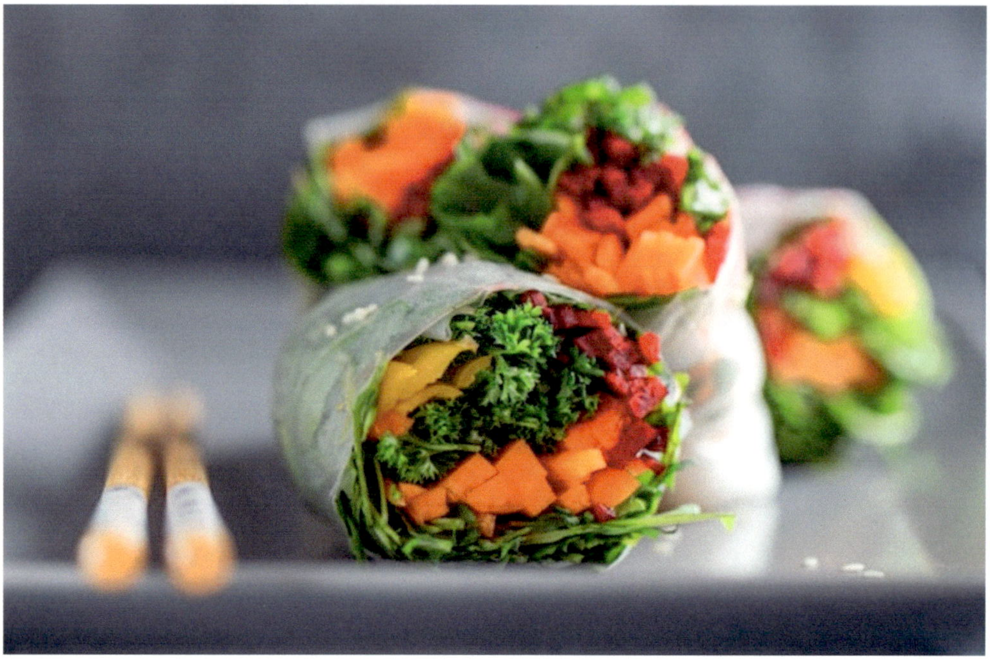

81. Veggie and Hummus Breakfast Wrap

Prep.Time: 5 min	Cook Time: 0 min	Serving: 1	Beverage pairing: Black Coffee

Ingredients:

- 1 whole wheat tortilla
- 2 tablespoons hummus
- 1/4 cup chopped mixed vegetables (such as bell peppers, cucumber, carrots)
- 1/4 cup baby spinach leaves
- 1 tablespoon crumbled feta cheese (optional)
- Salt and pepper to taste

Preparation:

1. Spread hummus evenly over the whole wheat tortilla.
2. Layer chopped mixed vegetables and baby spinach leaves on top of the hummus.
3. Sprinkle with crumbled feta cheese if desired.
4. Season with salt and pepper to taste.
5. Roll up the tortilla tightly to form a wrap.
6. Slice in half diagonally and serve.

Nutritional Facts (per serving):

- Calories: 200
- Carbohydrates: 25g
- Fat: 8g
- Protein: 6g

82. Vanilla Fig Protein Smoothie

Prep.Time:	Cook Time:	Serving:	Beverage pairing:
5 min	0 min	1	Herbal Tea

Ingredients:

- 1/2 cup unsweetened almond milk
- 1/2 cup Greek yogurt (unsweetened)
- 2 dried figs, chopped
- 1 scoop vanilla protein powder
- 1 tablespoon almond butter (unsweetened)
- Ice cubes (optional)

Preparation:

1. In a blender, combine unsweetened almond milk, Greek yogurt, dried figs, vanilla protein powder, and almond butter.
2. If desired, add ice cubes for a colder and thicker texture.
3. Blend until smooth and creamy.
4. Pour into a glass and serve immediately.

Nutritional Facts (per serving):

- Calories: 250
- Carbohydrates: 25g
- Fat: 10g
- Protein: 20g

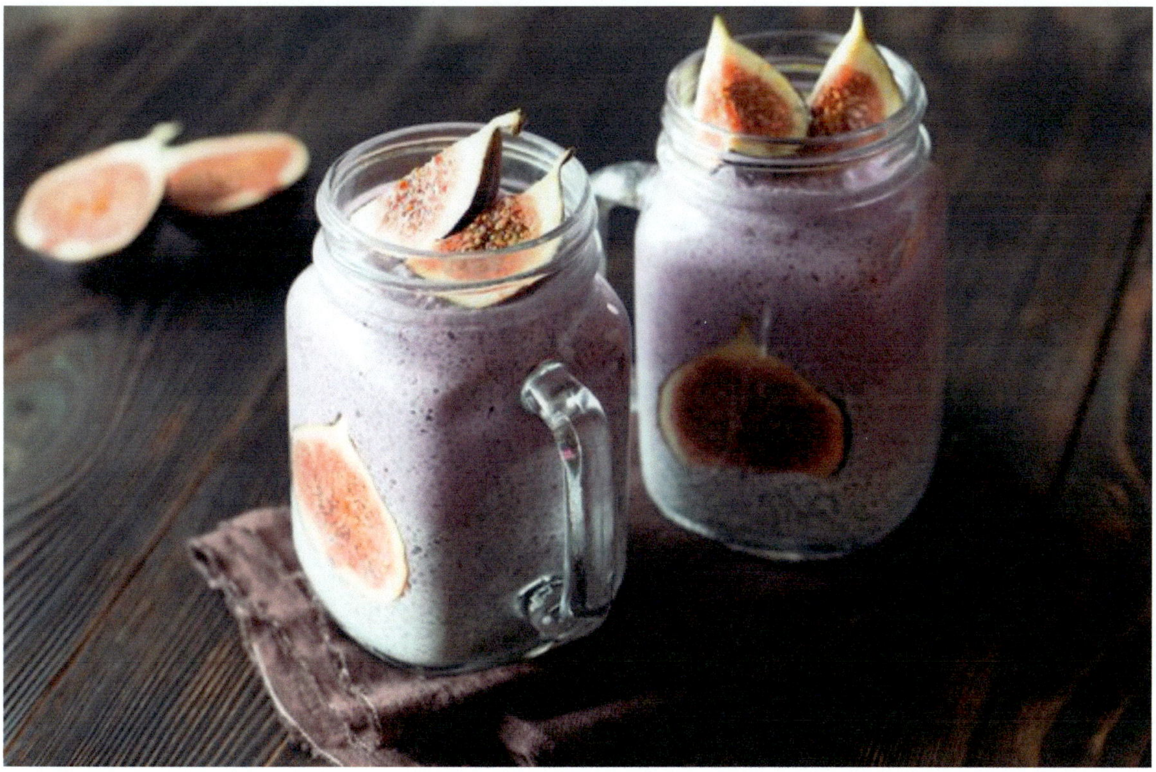

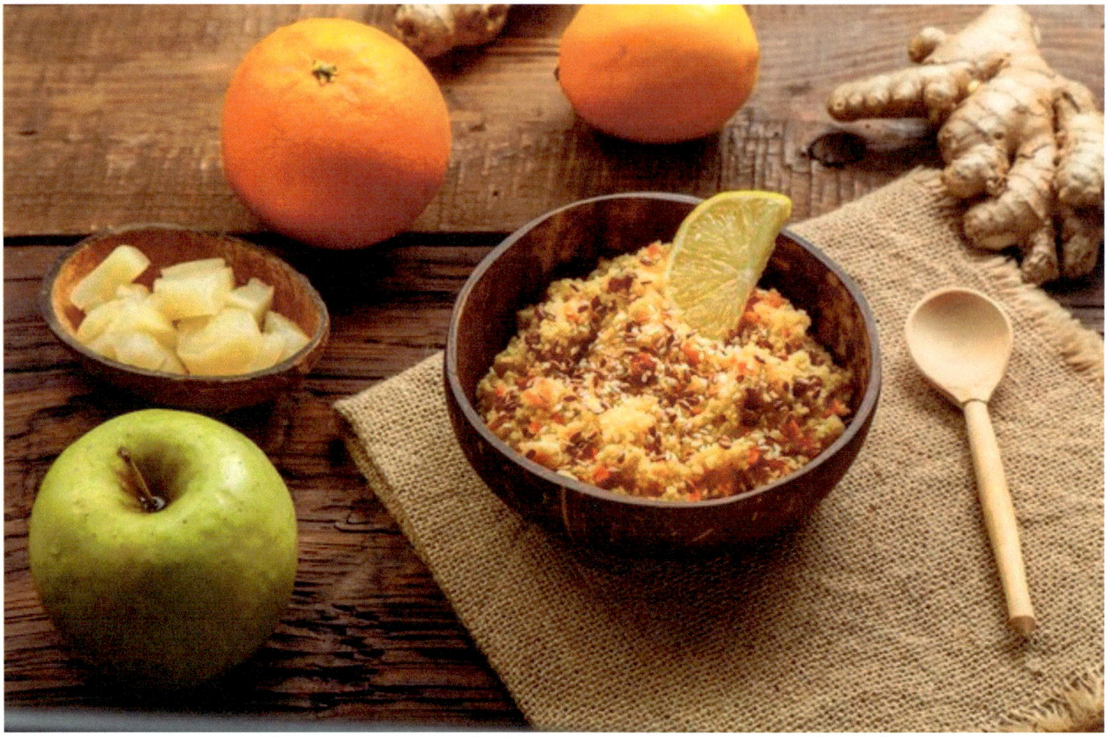

83. Apple Cider Quinoa Porridge

Prep.Time: 10 min

Cook Time: 0 min

Serving: 1

Beverage pairing: Black Coffee

Ingredients:

- 1/2 cup cooked quinoa
- 1/2 cup unsweetened apple cider
- 1/4 cup unsweetened applesauce
- 1 tablespoon chopped pecans
- 1/2 teaspoon ground cinnamon
- 1 teaspoon honey or maple syrup (optional)

Preparation:

1. In a small saucepan, combine cooked quinoa, unsweetened apple cider, unsweetened applesauce, chopped pecans, and ground cinnamon.
2. Cook over medium heat, stirring occasionally, until heated through and the mixture thickens to desired consistency.
3. If desired, sweeten with honey or maple syrup.
4. Remove from heat and serve warm.

Nutritional Facts (per serving):

- Calories: 250
- Carbohydrates: 40g
- Fat: 5g
- Protein: 5g

84. Caprese Egg Cups

Prep.Time:	Cook Time:	Serving:	Beverage pairing:
10 min	12-15 min	2	Herbal Tea

Ingredients:

- 4 large eggs
- 1/2 cup cherry tomatoes, halved
- 1/4 cup fresh mozzarella balls, halved
- 2 tablespoons chopped fresh basil
- Salt and pepper to taste

Preparation:

1. Preheat the oven to 375°F (190°C). Grease a muffin tin with cooking spray.
2. Crack one egg into each muffin cup.
3. Place cherry tomato halves and fresh mozzarella halves on top of each egg.
4. Sprinkle with chopped fresh basil.
5. Season with salt and pepper to taste.
6. Bake in the preheated oven for 12-15 minutes or until the egg whites are set and the yolks are cooked to your desired doneness.
7. Remove from the oven and let the egg cups cool slightly before serving.

Nutritional Facts (per serving - 2 egg cups):

- Calories: 200
- Carbohydrates: 5g
- Fat: 14g
- Protein: 15g

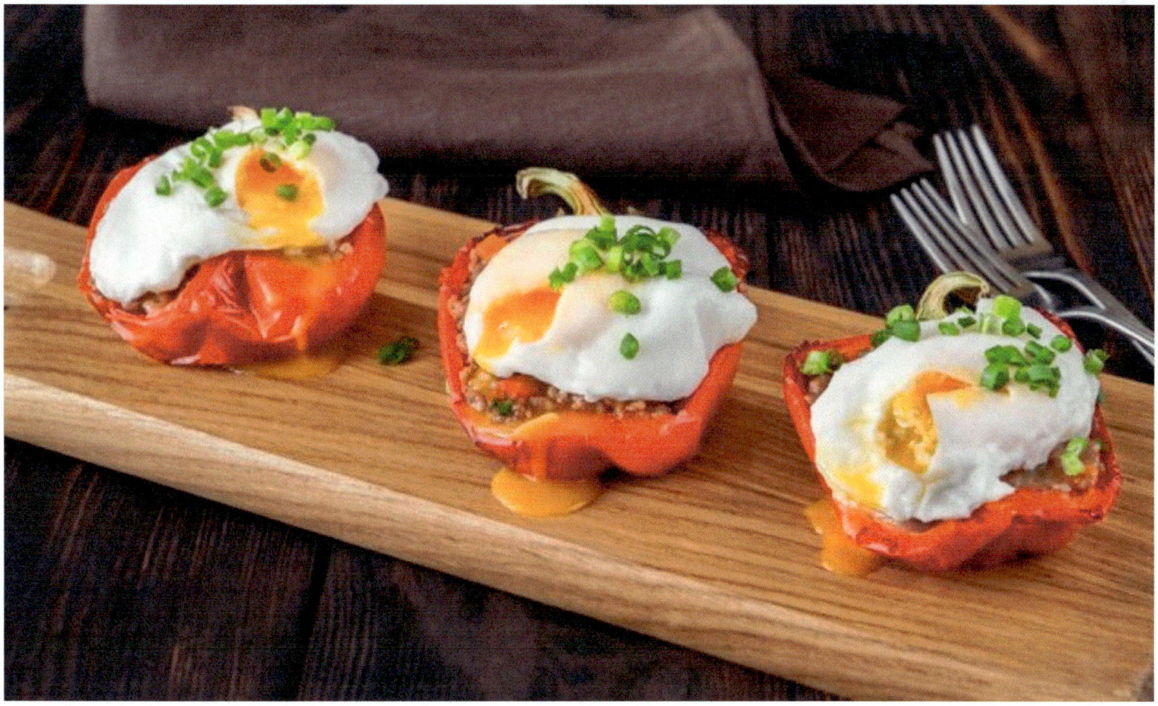

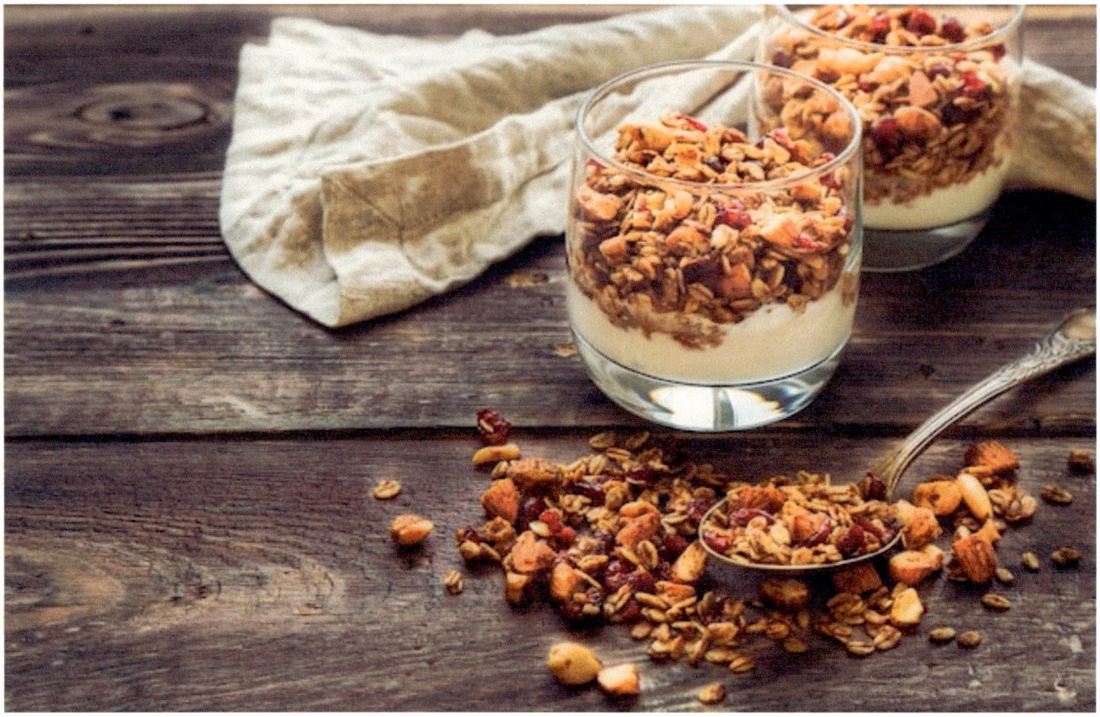

85. Pecan Pie Overnight Oats

Prep.Time: 5 min

Cook Time: 0 min

Serving: 1

Beverage pairing: Black Coffee

Ingredients:

- 1/2 cup rolled oats
- 1/2 cup unsweetened almond milk
- 1 tablespoon chopped pecans
- 1 tablespoon maple syrup
- 1/2 teaspoon vanilla extract
- Pinch of ground cinnamon
- Pinch of salt

Preparation:

1. In a jar or container, combine rolled oats, unsweetened almond milk, chopped pecans, maple syrup, vanilla extract, ground cinnamon, and salt.
2. Stir well to combine all ingredients.
3. Cover the jar/container and refrigerate overnight or for at least 4 hours.
4. In the morning, give the oats a stir and enjoy cold.

Nutritional Facts (per serving):

- Calories: 250
- Carbohydrates: 30g
- Fat: 10g
- Protein: 6g

86. Breakfast Stuffed Bell Peppers

Prep.Time: 15 min

Cook Time: 20-25 min

Serving: 4

Beverage pairing: Herbal Tea

Ingredients:

- 2 large bell peppers, halved and seeds removed
- 4 large eggs
- 1/2 cup cooked quinoa
- 1/4 cup diced tomatoes
- 1/4 cup diced onions
- 1/4 cup shredded cheddar cheese (reduced-fat)
- 1 tablespoon chopped fresh parsley
- Salt and pepper to taste

Preparation:

1. Preheat the oven to 375°F (190°C). Place the halved bell peppers in a baking dish.
2. In a bowl, whisk the eggs and season with salt and pepper.
3. Stir in cooked quinoa, diced tomatoes, diced onions, shredded cheddar cheese, and chopped fresh parsley.
4. Spoon the egg mixture into the bell pepper halves, filling them evenly.
5. Bake in the preheated oven for 20-25 minutes or until the eggs are set and the peppers are tender.
6. Remove from the oven and let them cool slightly before serving.

Nutritional Facts (per serving - 1 stuffed bell pepper half):

- Calories: 200
- Carbohydrates: 15g
- Fat: 10g
- Protein: 12g

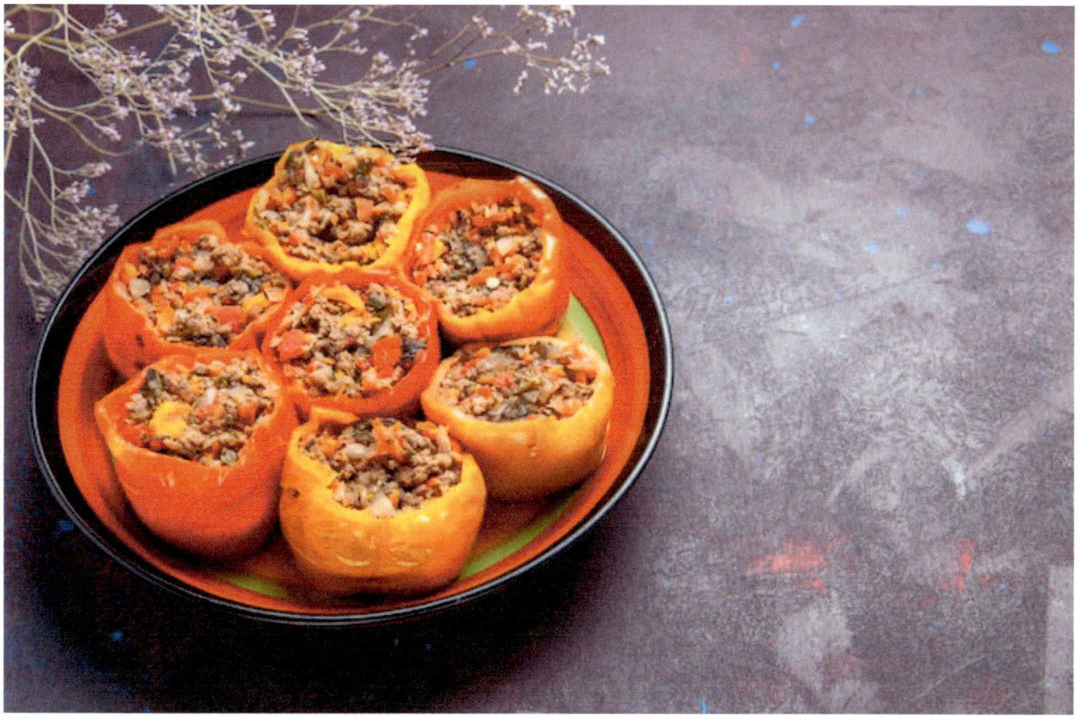

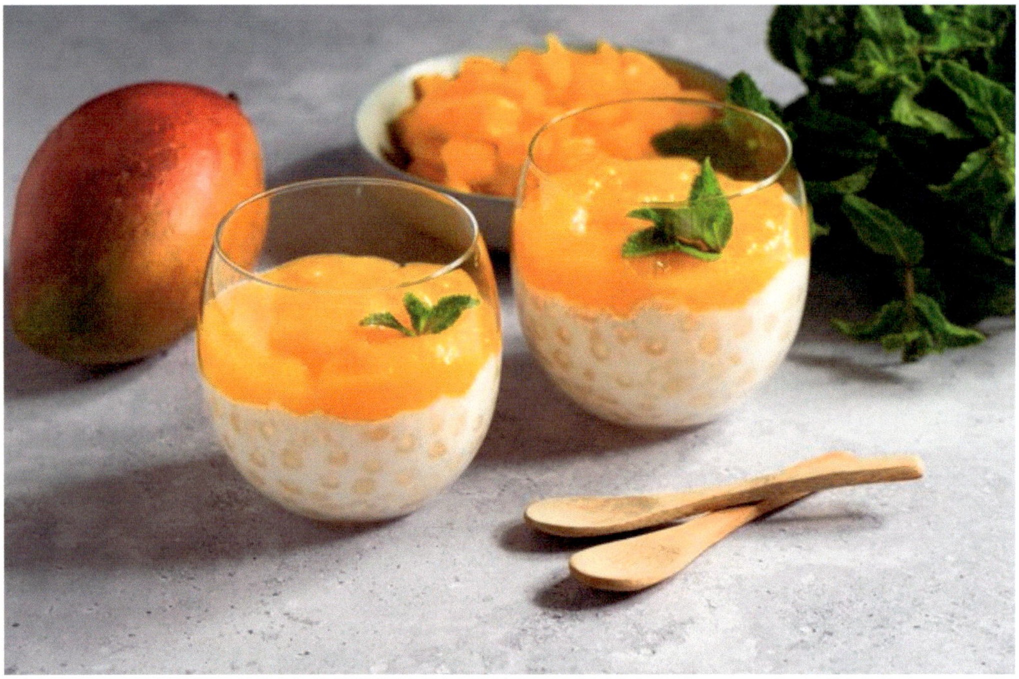

87. Mango Basil Yogurt Parfait

Prep.Time:	Cook Time:	Serving:	Beverage pairing:
5 min	0 min	1	Black Coffee

Ingredients:

- 1/2 cup Greek yogurt (unsweetened)
- 1/2 cup diced mango
- 2 tablespoons chopped fresh basil leaves
- 2 tablespoons granola (unsweetened)
- 1 tablespoon chopped nuts (almonds, walnuts, or pecans)
- 1 teaspoon honey or maple syrup (optional)

Preparation:

1. In a glass or parfait dish, layer Greek yogurt, diced mango, and chopped fresh basil leaves.
2. Sprinkle granola and chopped nuts on top of the yogurt and fruit layers.
3. Drizzle with honey or maple syrup if desired.
4. Repeat the layers until the glass is filled.
5. Serve immediately.

Nutritional Facts (per serving):

- Calories: 250
- Carbohydrates: 30g
- Fat: 10g
- Protein: 12g

88. Lemon Poppy Seed Pancakes

Prep.Time:	Cook Time:	Serving:	Beverage pairing:
10 min	10 min	4	Herbal Tea

Ingredients:

- 1 cup whole wheat flour
- 1 tablespoon poppy seeds
- 1 tablespoon lemon zest
- 1 tablespoon lemon juice
- 1 tablespoon honey or maple syrup
- 1 teaspoon baking powder
- 1/2 teaspoon baking soda
- 1 cup unsweetened almond milk
- 1 large egg
- Cooking spray

Preparation:

1. In a mixing bowl, combine whole wheat flour, poppy seeds, lemon zest, lemon juice, honey or maple syrup, baking powder, and baking soda.
2. In another bowl, whisk together unsweetened almond milk and egg.
3. Pour the wet ingredients into the dry ingredients and stir until just combined. Do not overmix; it's okay if the batter is slightly lumpy.
4. Heat a non-stick skillet over medium heat and lightly coat with cooking spray.
5. Pour about 1/4 cup of batter onto the skillet for each pancake.
6. Cook until bubbles form on the surface of the pancakes, then flip and cook until golden brown on both sides.
7. Repeat with the remaining batter.
8. Serve hot with your choice of toppings such as fresh berries or a drizzle of honey.

Nutritional Facts (per serving - 2 pancakes):

- Calories: 250
- Carbohydrates: 35g
- Fat: 8g
- Protein: 10g

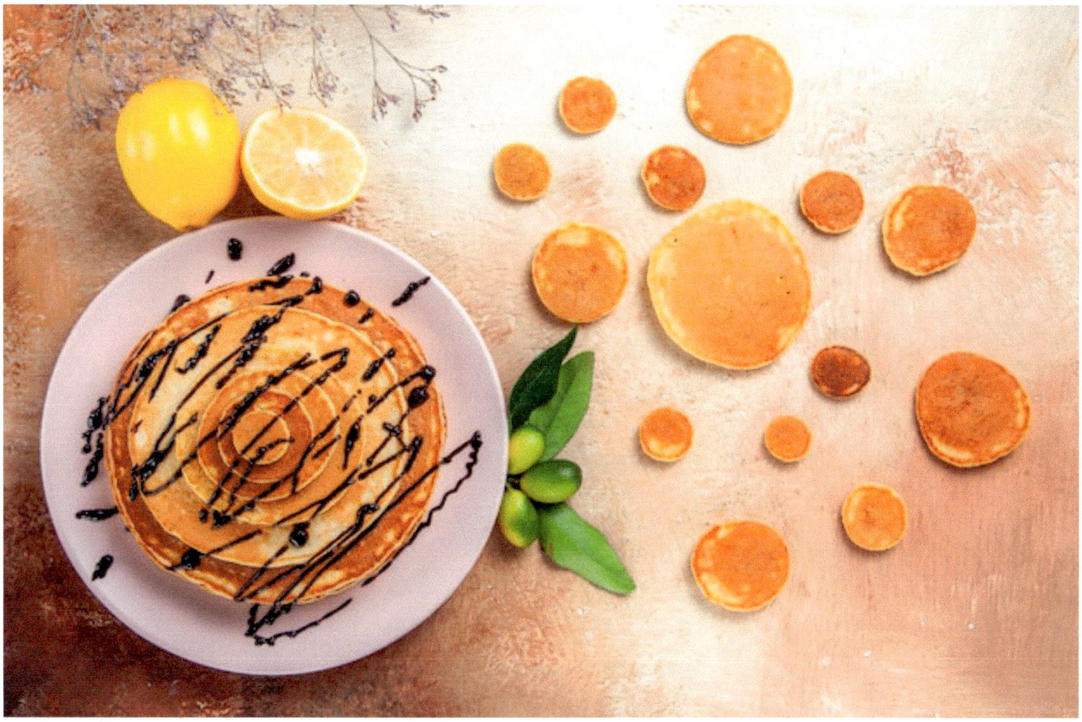

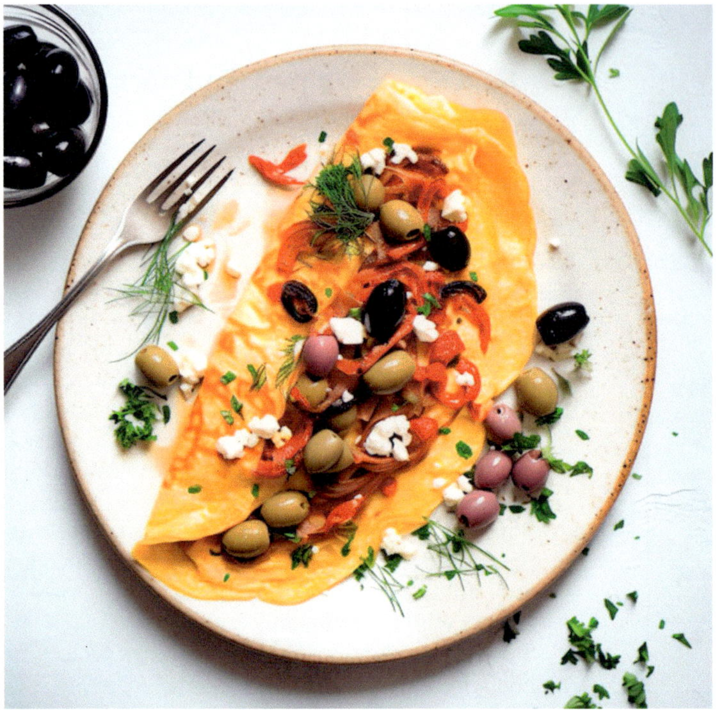

89. Greek Omelette with Olives and Feta

Prep.Time: 10 min | **Cook Time:** 5 min | **Serving:** 1 | **Beverage pairing:** Black Coffee

Ingredients:

- 2 large eggs
- 1/4 cup diced tomatoes
- 2 tablespoons diced red onions
- 2 tablespoons sliced black olives
- 2 tablespoons crumbled feta cheese
- 1 tablespoon chopped fresh parsley
- Salt and pepper to taste
- Cooking spray

Preparation:

1. In a bowl, beat the eggs and season with salt and pepper.
2. Heat a non-stick skillet over medium heat and lightly coat with cooking spray.
3. Pour the beaten eggs into the skillet and swirl to coat the bottom evenly.
4. Cook until the edges start to set, then use a spatula to gently lift the edges and let the uncooked eggs flow underneath.
5. Sprinkle diced tomatoes, diced red onions, sliced black olives, crumbled feta cheese, and chopped fresh parsley over one half of the omelette.
6. Fold the other half of the omelette over the filling.
7. Cook for another minute or until the eggs are fully set and the filling is warmed through.
8. Slide the omelette onto a plate and serve hot.

Nutritional Facts (per serving):

- Calories: 200
- Carbohydrates: 5g
- Fat: 15g
- Protein: 14g

90. Blueberry Banana Breakfast Burrito

Prep.Time: 5 min

Cook Time: 0 min

Serving: 1

Beverage pairing: Black Coffee

Ingredients:

- 1 whole wheat tortilla
- 1/2 banana, mashed
- 1/4 cup fresh blueberries
- 2 tablespoons Greek yogurt (unsweetened)
- 1 tablespoon almond butter (unsweetened)
- 1 teaspoon honey or maple syrup (optional)

Preparation:

1. Spread mashed banana evenly over the whole wheat tortilla.
2. Layer fresh blueberries on top of the mashed banana.
3. Spread Greek yogurt and almond butter over the blueberries.
4. Drizzle with honey or maple syrup if desired.
5. Roll up the tortilla tightly to form a burrito.
6. Slice in half diagonally and serve.

Nutritional Facts (per serving):

- Calories: 250
- Carbohydrates: 35g
- Fat: 8g
- Protein: 8g

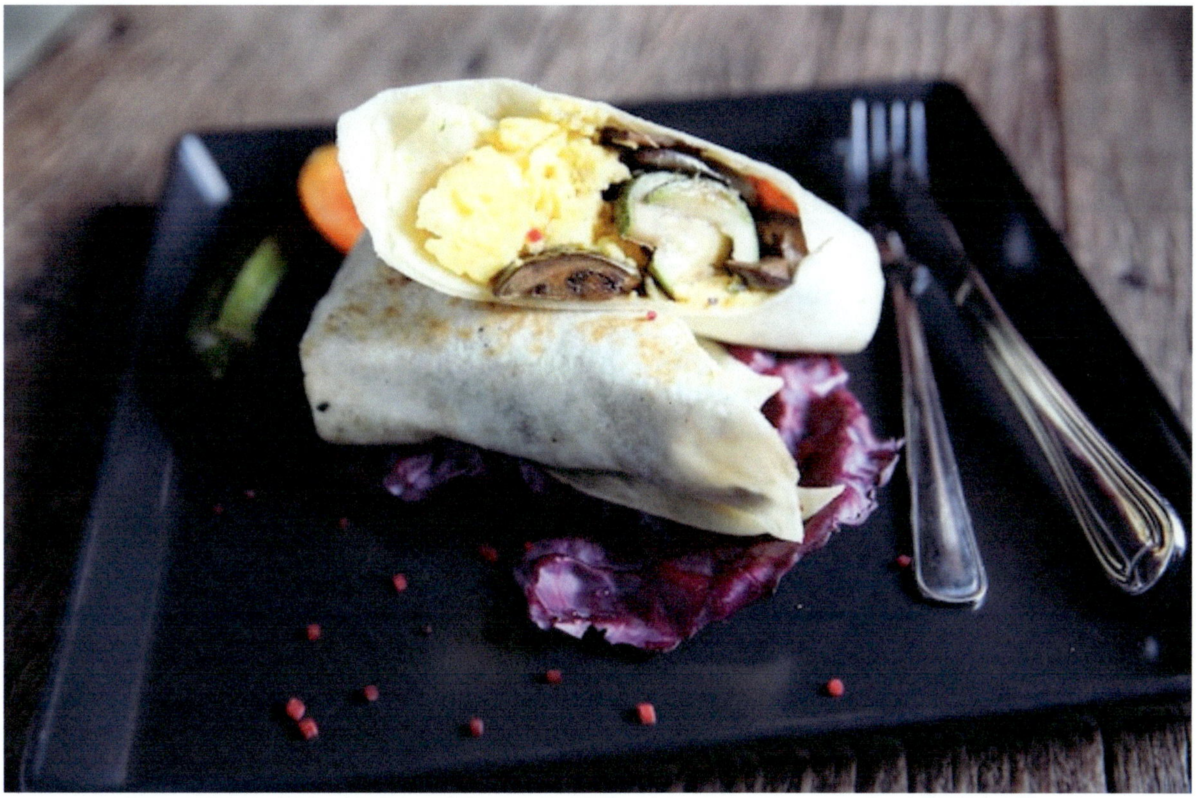

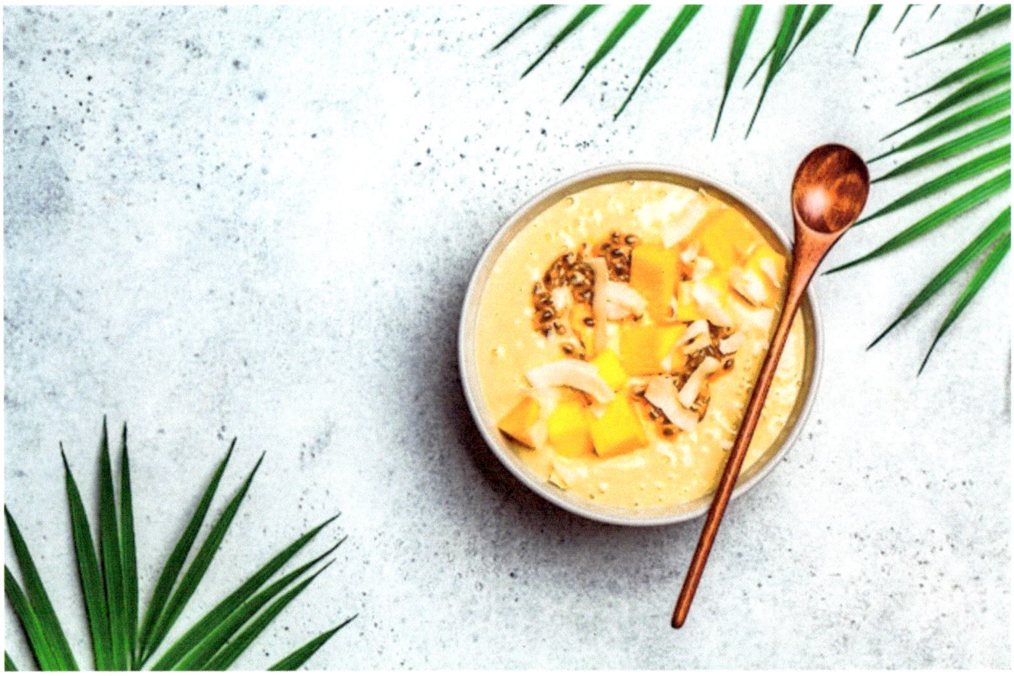

91. Coconut Mango Smoothie Bowl

Prep.Time: 5 min

Cook Time: 0 min

Serving: 1

Beverage pairing: Herbal Tea

Ingredients:

- 1/2 cup frozen mango chunks
- 1/2 banana
- 1/4 cup coconut milk
- 1/4 cup Greek yogurt (unsweetened)
- 2 tablespoons shredded coconut (unsweetened)
- 1 tablespoon chia seeds
- Fresh mango slices, for topping (optional)
- Fresh berries, for topping (optional)

Preparation:

1. In a blender, combine frozen mango chunks, banana, coconut milk, Greek yogurt, shredded coconut, and chia seeds.
2. Blend until smooth and creamy, adding more coconut milk if needed to reach desired consistency.
3. Pour the smoothie into a bowl.
4. Top with fresh mango slices and berries if desired.
5. Serve immediately.

Nutritional Facts (per serving):

- Calories: 300
- Carbohydrates: 30g
- Fat: 12g
- Protein: 10g

92. Pumpkin Walnut Breakfast Quinoa

Prep.Time: 10 min

Cook Time: 0 min

Serving: 1

Beverage pairing: Black Coffee

Ingredients:

- 1/2 cup cooked quinoa
- 1/4 cup canned pumpkin puree
- 2 tablespoons chopped walnuts
- 1 tablespoon maple syrup
- 1/2 teaspoon pumpkin pie spice
- 1/4 teaspoon vanilla extract
- Pinch of salt

Preparation:

1. In a small saucepan, combine cooked quinoa, canned pumpkin puree, chopped walnuts, maple syrup, pumpkin pie spice, vanilla extract, and a pinch of salt.
2. Cook over medium heat, stirring occasionally, until heated through and the flavors are well combined.
3. Remove from heat and serve warm.

Nutritional Facts (per serving):

- Calories: 250
- Carbohydrates: 30g
- Fat: 10g
- Protein: 6g

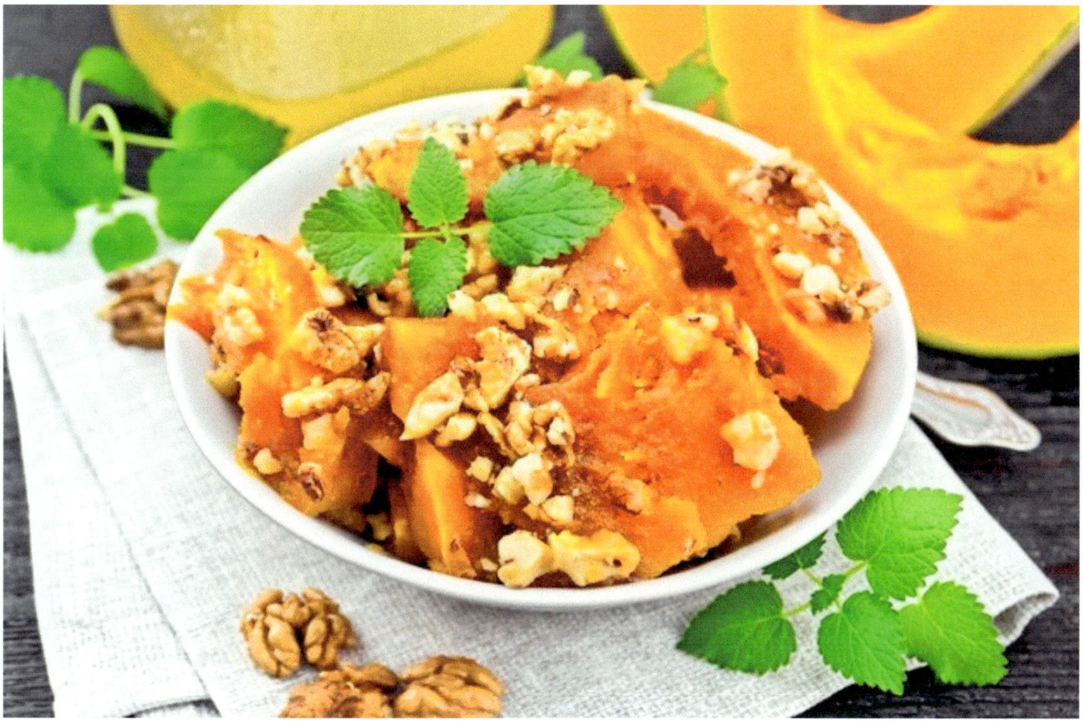

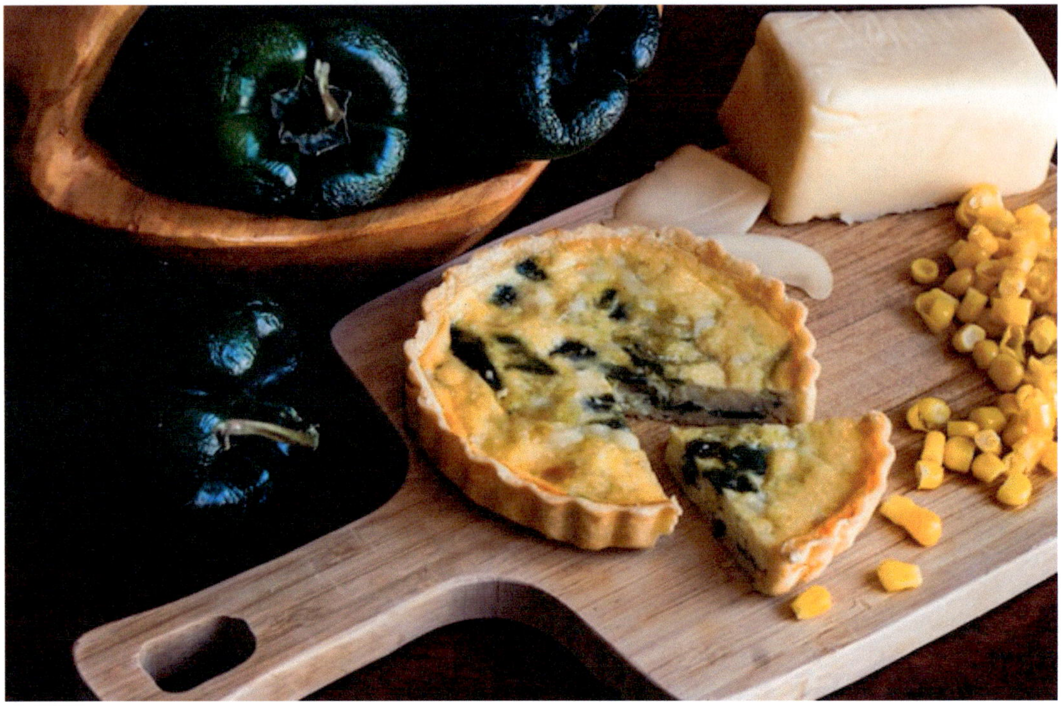

93. Spinach and Artichoke Quiche

Prep.Time: 15 min	**Cook Time:** 35-40 min	**Serving:** 6	**Beverage pairing:** Herbal Tea

Ingredients:

- 1 pie crust (store-bought or homemade)
- 4 large eggs
- 1 cup milk (any type)
- 1 cup chopped fresh spinach
- 1/2 cup chopped artichoke hearts (canned or cooked)
- 1/2 cup shredded mozzarella cheese
- 1/4 cup grated Parmesan cheese
- 2 cloves garlic, minced
- 1 tablespoon olive oil
- Salt and pepper to taste

Preparation:

1. Preheat the oven to 375°F (190°C). Place the pie crust in a pie dish and set aside.
2. In a skillet, heat olive oil over medium heat. Add minced garlic and sauté until fragrant.
3. Add chopped spinach and chopped artichoke hearts to the skillet. Cook until the spinach wilts and the artichokes are heated through. Remove from heat and let it cool slightly.
4. In a mixing bowl, whisk together eggs and milk. Season with salt and pepper.
5. Stir in the cooked spinach and artichoke mixture, shredded mozzarella cheese, and grated Parmesan cheese.
6. Pour the mixture into the prepared pie crust.
7. Bake in the preheated oven for 35-40 minutes or until the quiche is set and the crust is golden brown.
8. Remove from the oven and let it cool for a few minutes before slicing and serving.

Nutritional Facts (per serving):

- Calories: 300
- Carbohydrates: 20g
- Fat: 18g
- Protein: 14g

94. Almond Joy Chia Pudding

Prep.Time: 5 min | **Cook Time:** 0 min | **Serving:** 1 | **Beverage pairing:** Black Coffee

Ingredients:

- 1/4 cup chia seeds
- 1 cup unsweetened almond milk
- 2 tablespoons unsweetened shredded coconut
- 1 tablespoon cocoa powder
- 1 tablespoon almond butter (unsweetened)
- 1 tablespoon maple syrup
- 1/4 teaspoon almond extract
- 1/4 cup sliced almonds (optional, for garnish)

Preparation:

1. In a jar or container, combine chia seeds, unsweetened almond milk, shredded coconut, cocoa powder, almond butter, maple syrup, and almond extract.
2. Stir well to combine all ingredients.
3. Cover the jar/container and refrigerate overnight or for at least 4 hours, allowing the chia seeds to gel and thicken.
4. Before serving, give the pudding a stir.
5. Garnish with sliced almonds if desired.

Nutritional Facts (per serving):

- Calories: 250
- Carbohydrates: 20g
- Fat: 15g
- Protein: 7g

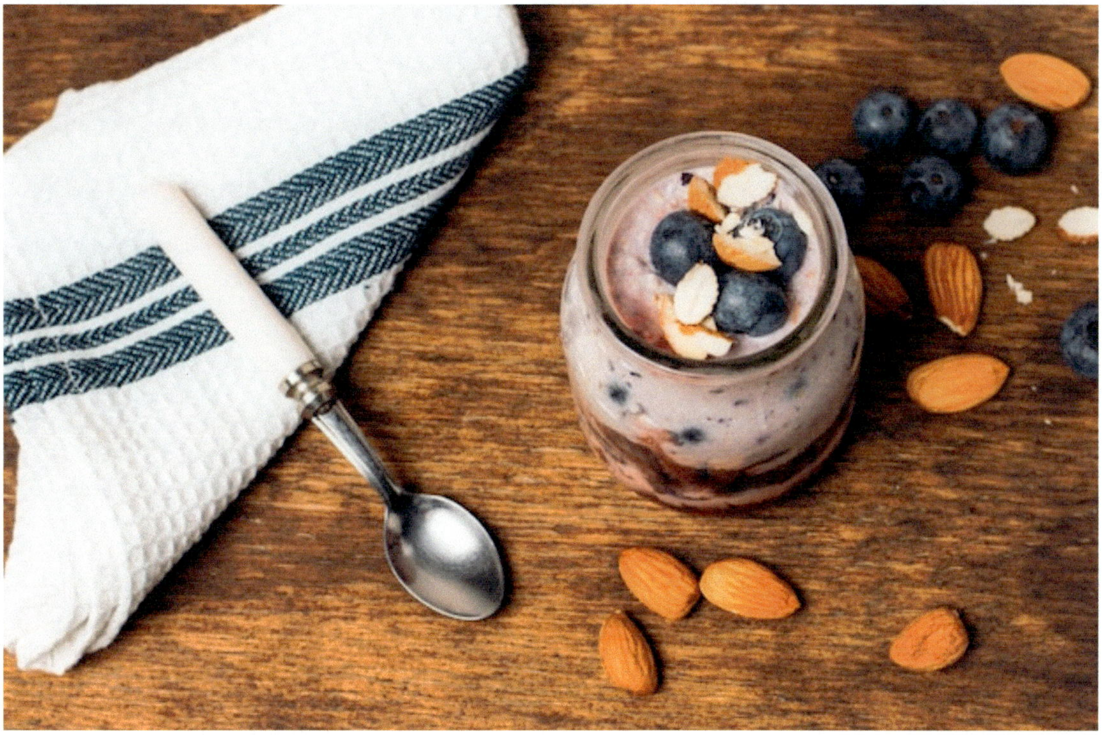

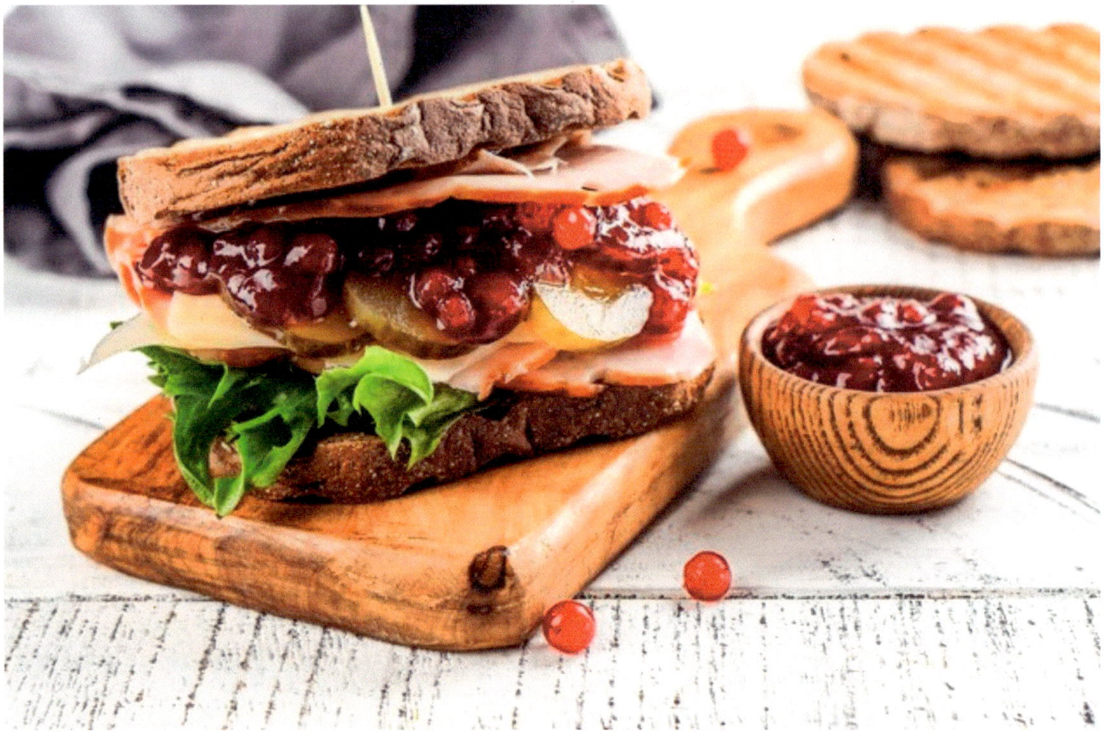

95. Turkey and Cranberry Breakfast Sandwich

Prep.Time:	Cook Time:	Serving:	Beverage pairing:
10 min	0 min	1	Herbal Tea

Ingredients:

- 1 whole wheat English muffin, split and toasted
- 2 slices turkey bacon
- 1 large egg
- 1 tablespoon cranberry sauce
- 1 teaspoon Dijon mustard
- Salt and pepper to taste
- Cooking spray

Preparation:

1. Cook turkey bacon according to package instructions until crispy. Set aside.
2. Heat a non-stick skillet over medium heat and lightly coat with cooking spray.
3. Crack the egg into the skillet and cook to your desired doneness. Season with salt and pepper.
4. Spread cranberry sauce on one half of the toasted English muffin and Dijon mustard on the other half.
5. Layer cooked turkey bacon and the fried egg on one half of the English muffin.
6. Top with the other half of the English muffin to make a sandwich.
7. Serve immediately.

Nutritional Facts (per serving):

- Calories: 250
- Carbohydrates: 25g
- Fat: 10g
- Protein: 15g

96. Chocolate Raspberry Protein Pancakes

Prep.Time: 10 min

Cook Time: 10 min

Serving: 4

Beverage pairing: Herbal Tea

Ingredients:

- 1/2 cup whole wheat flour
- 1 scoop chocolate protein powder
- 1 teaspoon baking powder
- 1/4 teaspoon salt
- 1/2 cup unsweetened almond milk
- 1 large egg
- 1 tablespoon cocoa powder
- 1/4 cup fresh raspberries
- Cooking spray

Preparation:

1. In a mixing bowl, whisk together whole wheat flour, chocolate protein powder, baking powder, and salt.
2. In another bowl, whisk together unsweetened almond milk, egg, and cocoa powder until well combined.
3. Pour the wet ingredients into the dry ingredients and stir until just combined. Do not overmix; it's okay if the batter is slightly lumpy.
4. Gently fold in fresh raspberries.
5. Heat a non-stick skillet or griddle over medium heat and lightly coat with cooking spray.
6. Pour about 1/4 cup of batter onto the skillet for each pancake.
7. Cook until bubbles form on the surface of the pancakes, then flip and cook until golden brown on both sides.
8. Repeat with the remaining batter.
9. Serve hot with additional fresh raspberries on top if desired.

Nutritional Facts (per serving - 2 pancakes):

- Calories: 300
- Carbohydrates: 25g
- Fat: 8g
- Protein: 20g

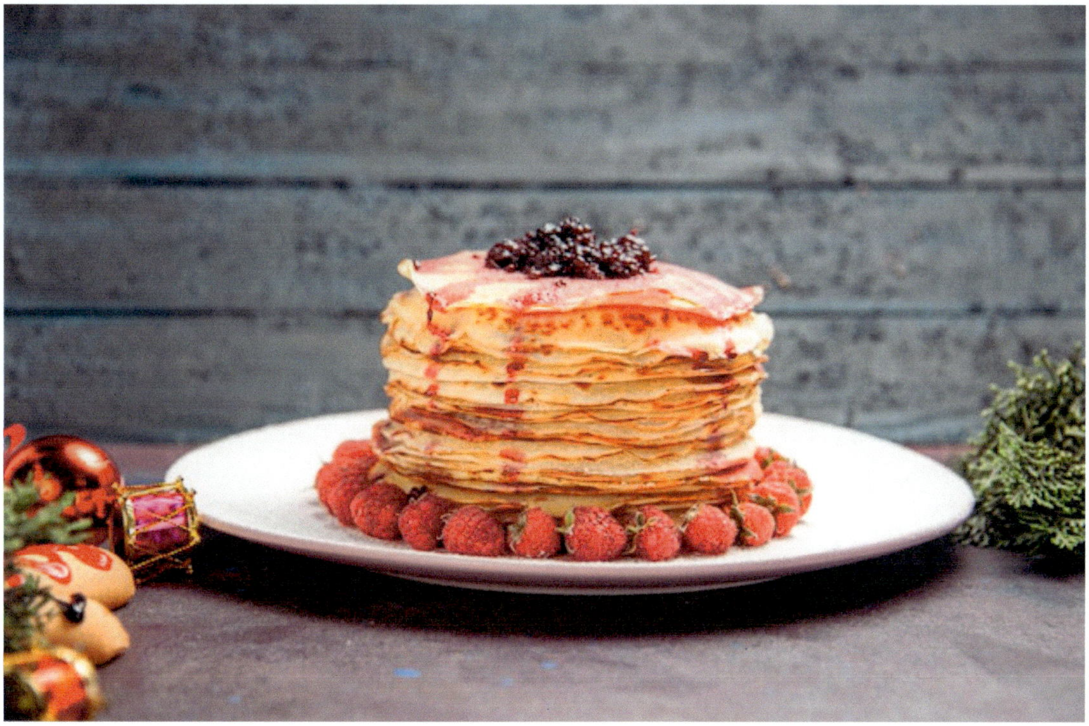

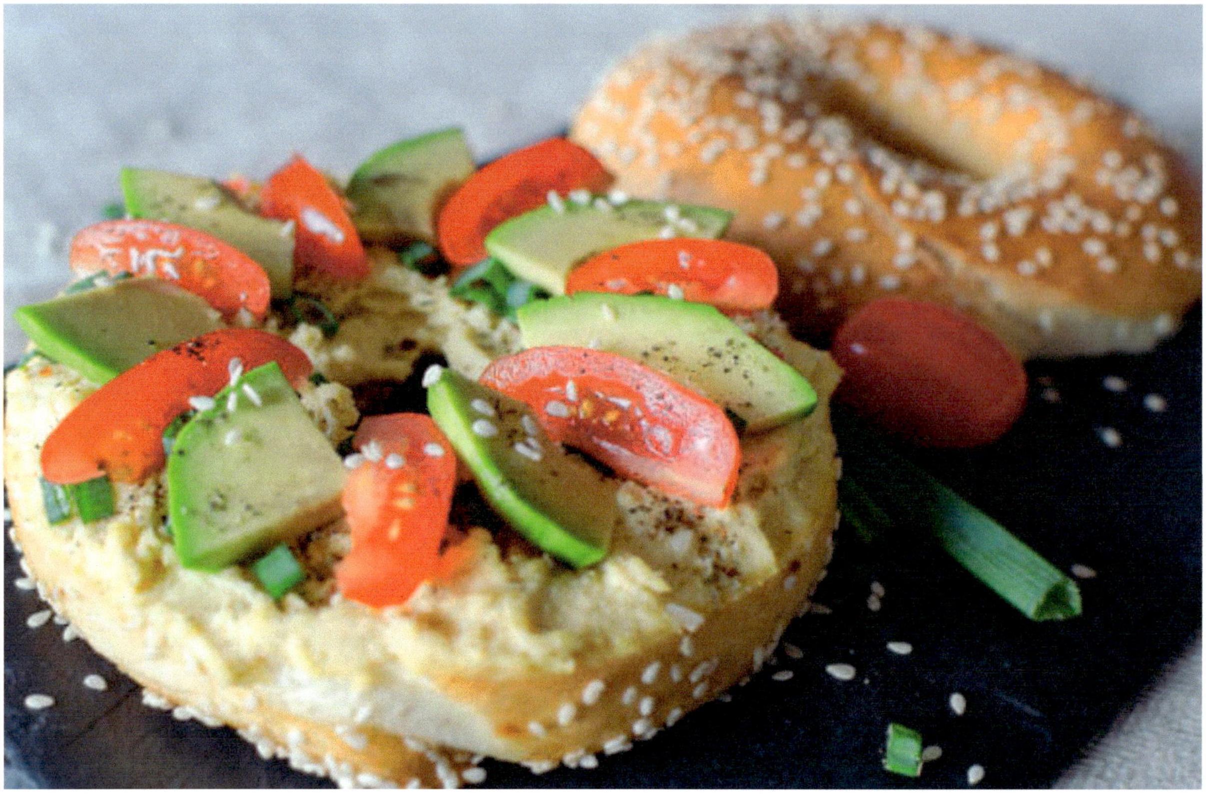

97. Avocado and Cherry Tomato Bagel

Prep.Time:	Cook Time:	Serving:	Beverage pairing:
5 min	0 min	1	Black Coffee

Ingredients:

- 1 whole grain bagel, split and toasted
- 1/2 avocado, mashed
- 1/4 cup cherry tomatoes, halved
- Salt and pepper to taste

Preparation:

1. Spread mashed avocado evenly on both halves of the toasted whole grain bagel.
2. Top with halved cherry tomatoes.
3. Season with salt and pepper to taste.
4. Serve immediately.

Nutritional Facts (per serving):

- Calories: 250
- Carbohydrates: 30g
- Fat: 10g
- Protein: 8g

98. Peach Almond Breakfast Couscous

Prep.Time:	Cook Time:	Serving:	Beverage pairing:
10 min	10 min	4	Herbal Tea

Ingredients:

- 1/2 cup dry couscous
- 1/2 cup unsweetened almond milk
- 1/2 cup chopped peaches (fresh or frozen)
- 2 tablespoons sliced almonds
- 1 tablespoon honey or maple syrup
- 1/4 teaspoon almond extract

Preparation:

1. In a small saucepan, bring unsweetened almond milk to a boil.
2. Stir in dry couscous, reduce heat to low, cover, and simmer for 5 minutes or until the couscous is cooked and has absorbed the liquid.
3. Fluff the cooked couscous with a fork.
4. Stir in chopped peaches, sliced almonds, honey or maple syrup, and almond extract.
5. Serve warm.

Nutritional Facts (per serving):

- Calories: 250
- Carbohydrates: 40g
- Fat: 6g
- Protein: 6g

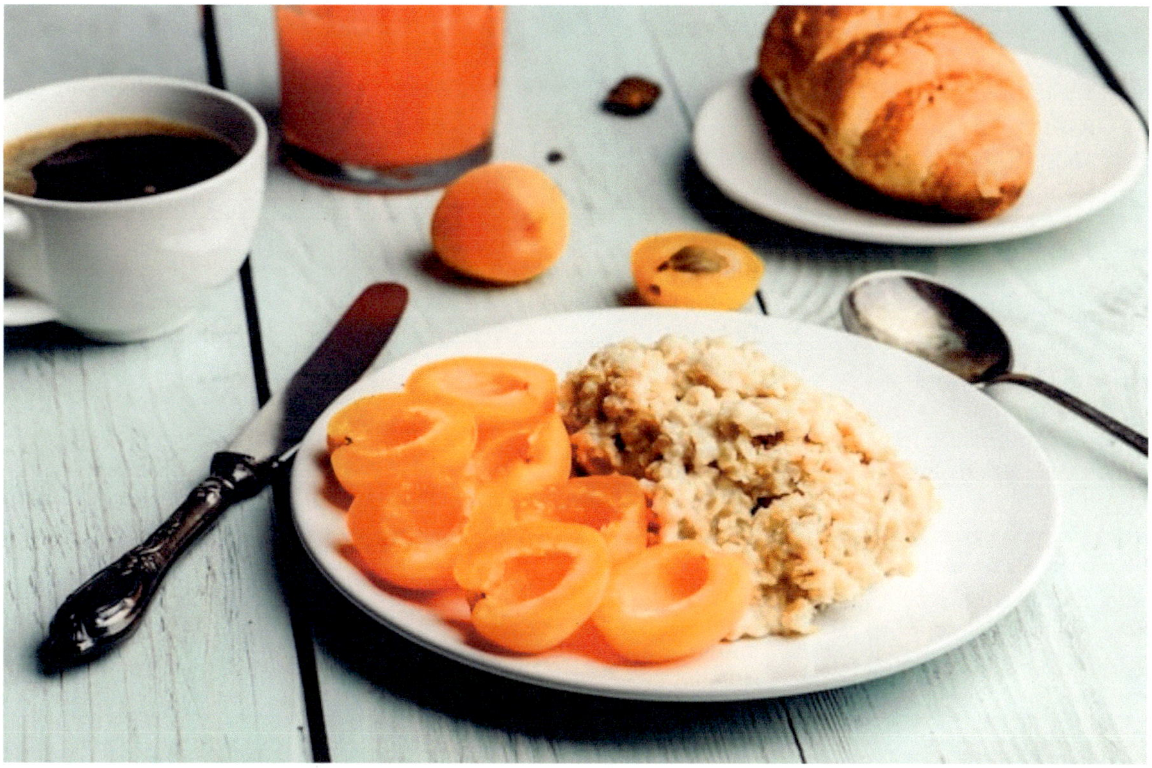

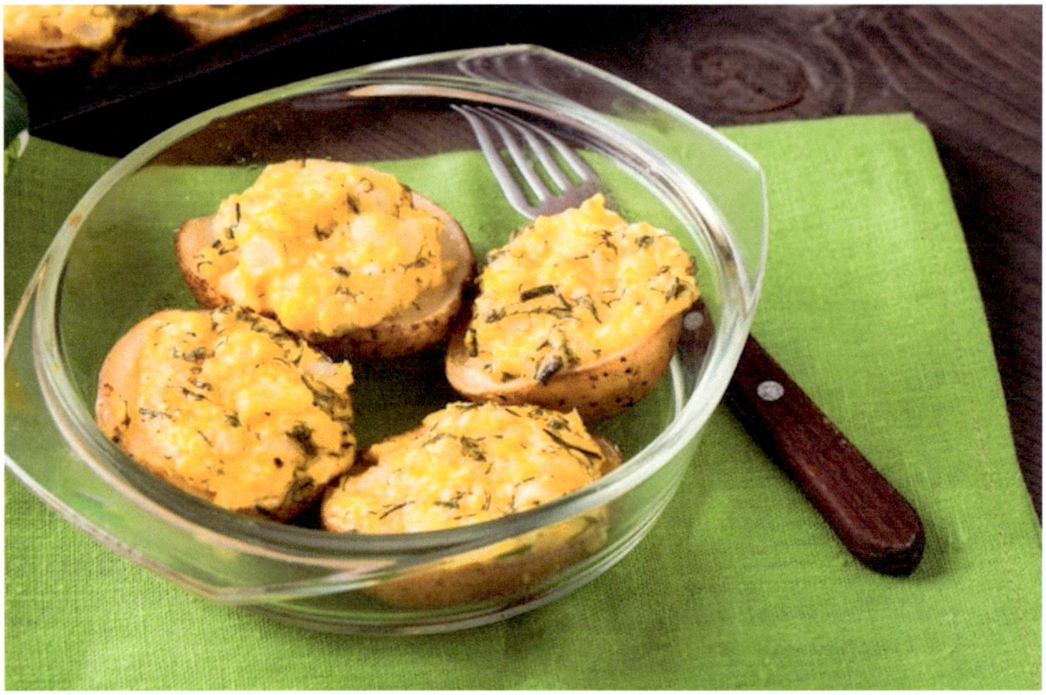

99. Broccoli and Cheddar Breakfast Muffins

Prep.Time: 10 min

Cook Time: 18-20 min

Serving: 12

Beverage pairing: Black Coffee

Ingredients:

- 1 cup whole wheat flour
- 1 teaspoon baking powder
- 1/2 teaspoon baking soda
- 1/4 teaspoon salt
- 2 large eggs
- 1/2 cup unsweetened almond milk
- 1/4 cup Greek yogurt (unsweetened)
- 1 tablespoon olive oil
- 1 cup chopped broccoli florets
- 1/2 cup shredded cheddar cheese
- Cooking spray

Preparation:

1. Preheat the oven to 375°F (190°C). Grease a muffin tin with cooking spray or line with paper liners.
2. In a large mixing bowl, whisk together whole wheat flour, baking powder, baking soda, and salt.
3. In another bowl, beat the eggs, then stir in unsweetened almond milk, Greek yogurt, and olive oil until well combined.
4. Pour the wet ingredients into the dry ingredients and mix until just combined.
5. Fold in chopped broccoli florets and shredded cheddar cheese.
6. Divide the batter evenly among the muffin cups, filling each about 3/4 full.
7. Bake in the preheated oven for 18-20 minutes or until a toothpick inserted into the center comes out clean.
8. Remove from the oven and let the muffins cool in the tin for a few minutes before transferring to a wire rack to cool completely.

Nutritional Facts (per muffin):

- Calories: 150
- Carbohydrates: 15g
- Fat: 7g
- Protein: 8g

100. Kiwi Lime Overnight Oats

Prep.Time: 5 min	**Cook Time:** 0 min	**Serving:** 1	**Beverage pairing:** Herbal Tea

Ingredients:

- 1/2 cup rolled oats
- 1/2 cup unsweetened almond milk
- 1 kiwi, peeled and diced
- Zest and juice of 1 lime
- 1 tablespoon honey or maple syrup (optional)
- Sliced kiwi and lime wedges, for garnish (optional)

Preparation:

1. In a jar or container, combine rolled oats, unsweetened almond milk, diced kiwi, lime zest, lime juice, and honey or maple syrup if using.
2. Stir well to combine all ingredients.
3. Cover the jar/container and refrigerate overnight or for at least 4 hours.
4. In the morning, give the oats a stir.
5. Garnish with sliced kiwi and lime wedges if desired before serving.

Nutritional Facts (per serving):

- Calories: 250
- Carbohydrates: 40g
- Fat: 5g
- Protein: 8g

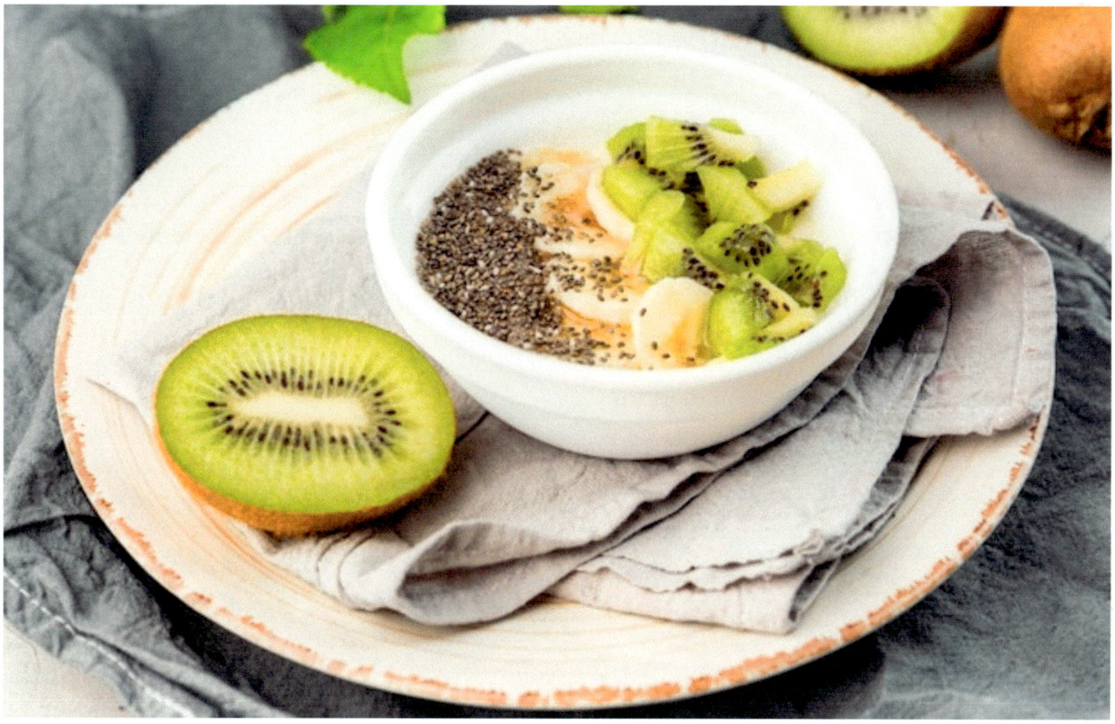

Sharing Your Culinary Journey

Now that you've mastered the art of creating delicious, diabetes-friendly meals, it's time to share your newfound culinary wisdom with others who are on the same path. By leaving your honest review of the "Type 2 Diabetes Cookbook: Beginner's Quick & Easy Recipes for Delicious Diabetes Diets" by Lily Anders on Amazon, you'll guide fellow food enthusiasts to a resource that can transform their dining table and health.

Your insights and experiences are invaluable, offering a beacon to those navigating their diet amidst diabetes. Whether it was a specific recipe that became your go-to, a tip that changed how you approach cooking, or the overall ease and enjoyment you found in these pages, your feedback is a gift that keeps on giving.

Thank you for contributing to a community of knowledge and support. The journey towards healthy eating and diabetes management thrives on shared discoveries and successes. By passing on your review, you're not just recommending a book—you're enriching lives with the joy of cooking and the empowerment of dietary control.

To leave your review, just follow this link:

https://www.amazon.com/review/create-review/?ie=UTF8&channel=glance-detail&asin=1963939298

Together, we're keeping the passion for healthy, joyful eating alive, one review at a time. Your support makes all the difference, not just to us, but to every reader and cook who seeks to balance their love for food with their health needs.

- With heartfelt thanks,

Lily Anders

Conclusion

In conclusion, this book transcends the traditional approach to managing diabetes through diet alone, offering a comprehensive guide that empowers individuals with diabetes to navigate their condition with knowledge and precision. Through 300 carefully crafted recipes, we explore the importance of balancing nutrient intake and the vital role of consistent meal planning. Each recipe is not just a set of instructions but a building block towards a healthier life, tailored to the unique needs of those managing diabetes.

As we close this journey of understanding and adaptation, remember that managing diabetes is not just about adhering to dietary restrictions or grappling with numbers—it is about reclaiming control of your health and life. These recipes are designed not only to meet specific nutritional needs but also to delight the palate, proving that a diabetes-conscious diet can be as delicious as it is nutritious.

Embrace these culinary tools as your allies in the pursuit of wellness. Let each meal enrich your body and spirit, and may the knowledge contained in this book guide you toward a balanced, joyful, and healthy life with diabetes. Here's to finding pleasure in every bite and strength in every challenge. Cheers to your health and happiness on this flavorful journey!

Made in the USA
Columbia, SC
18 September 2026

3f9d74e6-ce4b-4922-8aa2-6c42a0512ae8R01